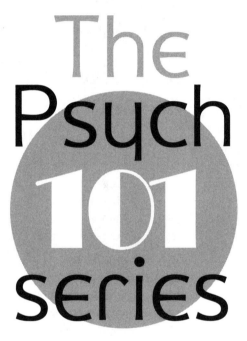

James C. Kaufman, PhD, Series Editor
Director, Learning Research Institute
California State University at San Bernardino

Lauren M. Rossen obtained her MS in Clinical and Health Psychology from the University of Florida and is currently a doctoral candidate in the Health Policy and Management program at the Johns Hopkins Bloomberg School of Public Health. She has been integrally involved in research that examined various methods of behavioral weight-loss treatment both at the University of Pennsylvania and at the University of Florida and has also worked directly with obese adolescents and adults undergoing weight-loss surgery. She has published numerous manuscripts on a variety of topics related to obesity, including psychosocial factors pertaining to cosmetic surgery, body image issues and related clinical disorders, psychosocial impacts of obesity and weight-loss treatment, dieting histories among bariatric surgery candidates, long-term outcomes of behavioral weight-loss treatments, and environmental factors related to physical activity behaviors among children. Her current research interests focus on factors contributing to childhood obesity and public health policy issues pertaining to obesity prevention.

Dr. Eric A. Rossen holds a PhD in School Psychology from the University of Florida and is a nationally certified school psychologist and licensed psychologist in the state of Maryland. He has experience working in public schools as well as in independent practice and is currently the Director of Professional Development and Standards for the National Association of School Psychologists. Aside from his interests in the psychosocial impacts of obesity, Dr. Rossen has published several manuscripts and presented nationally on issues related to bullying, crisis response, behavior management, emotional intelligence, and psychological assessment. He has also served as a college instructor and adjunct faculty at the University of Florida, University of Missouri, and Prince George's Community College.

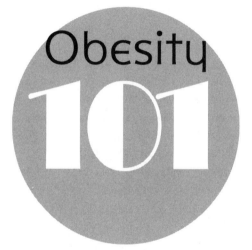

Obesity 101

Lauren M. Rossen, MS

Eric A. Rossen, PhD

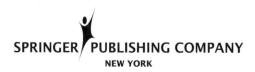

SPRINGER PUBLISHING COMPANY
NEW YORK

Copyright © 2012 Springer Publishing Company, LLC

Springer Publishing Company, LLC
11 West 42nd Street
New York, NY 10036
www.springerpub.com

Acquisitions Editor: Nancy Hale
Composition: Newgen Imaging

ISBN: 978-0-8261-0744-2
E-book ISBN: 978-0-8261-0745-9

11 12 13 / 5 4 3 2 1

Library of Congress Cataloging-in-Publication Data
Rossen, Lauren M.
    Obesity 101 / Lauren M. Rossen & Eric A. Rossen.
      p. ; cm. — (Psych 101 series)
    Obesity one hundred one
    Obesity one hundred and one
    Includes bibliographical references and index.
    ISBN 978-0-8261-0744-2 — ISBN 978-0-8261-0745-9 (e-book)
    1. Obesity. I. Rossen, Eric A. II. Title. III. Title: Obesity one hundred one. IV. Title:
Obesity one hundred and one. V. Series: Psych 101 series.
    [DNLM: 1. Obesity. WD 210]
    RC628.R66 2012
    616.3'98—dc23   2011027053

Printed in the United States of America by Hamilton Printing

To our beautiful daughter, Emily,
who in a short time has taught us humility, patience,
and perspective.
May you derive as much pleasure from life as we
have from watching you grow.

And to Layla,
for your unwavering loyalty
and willingness to keep us company during
long sessions in front of the computer.
You're a good dog.

Contents

Creativity 101
James C. Kaufman, PhD

Genius 101
Dean Keith Simonton, PhD

IQ Testing 101
Alan S. Kaufman, PhD

Leadership 101
Michael D. Mumford, PhD

Psycholinguistics 101
H. Wind Cowles, PhD

Anxiety 101
Moshe Zeidner, PhD
Gerald Matthews, PhD

Humor 101
Mitch Earleywine, PhD

Obesity 101
Lauren M. Rossen, MS
Eric A. Rossen, PhD

Emotional Intelligence 101
Gerald Matthews, PhD
Moshe Zeidner, PhD
Richard D. Roberts, PhD

Intelligence 101
Jonathan Plucker, PhD

Introduction

hances are, if you have watched more than 30 seconds of television (TV) or glanced at a newspaper or magazine within the past 24 hours, you've seen a story about obesity, which always seems to include a clip of some unwitting overweight pedestrian's backside, shown from the neck down. At the very least, you have seen commercials for the latest weight-loss product, which always seem to include a "before" and "after" shot of what can only be two entirely different people wearing the same outfit. Coverage of obesity in the popular press has reached a fever pitch in recent years. In fact, the number of news articles mentioning obesity has skyrocketed, from a total of 429 in 1980, to 14,514 in 2000, to more than 3,000 in a single day in January 2010 (that would mean more than 93,000 for just 1 month; see Figure 1.1).

So why is America obsessed with the topic of obesity and weight loss? What exactly is obesity? And perhaps most importantly, what can we do about it?

1

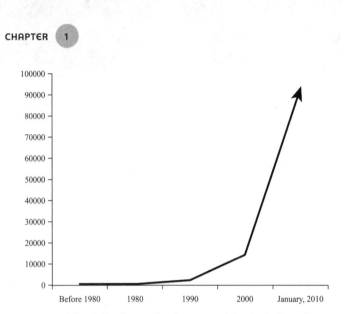

FIGURE 1.1 A LexisNexis search of news articles including the term obesity from prior to 1980–2010.

WHAT IS OBESITY?

Defining obesity is sort of like defining who can or can't ride on a roller coaster. If you've been to an amusement park, you probably recall seeing signs saying, "must be *this tall* to ride" next to a cardboard cartoon character about 40 inches tall. Surely, these signs exist not to frustrate hundreds of children who are short for their age, but for some safety-related reason. Perhaps the ride is too scary for young children, so the height requirement is designed to weed out those kids too young to ride. But if that is the case, then why have a height requirement at all? Why not just get children's ages? After all, that may not be fair to adults who are actually shorter than the height minimum. Well, that may be difficult, since not many children walk around with copies of their birth certificates at the ready in case someone needs to verify their ages.

Maybe the ride would be unsafe for small children because they are too light, and the safety restraints would not be tight enough to hold them in place. But in that case, why not get children's weights or waist circumferences to make sure the seatbelts will fit? Again, that presents some issues. You could ask children (or their parents) what they weigh, but are you confident that their responses would be accurate? A better way would be to actually measure their weights or waist circumferences, but that hardly seems practical. Those 2-hour lines for Space Mountain would stretch to 4 hours if each child had to be weighed and measured before riding. So in the end, maybe having a simple sign, "must be *this tall* to ride" is the easiest way to ensure safety, even if it is unfair to all those kids who are just a little short for their ages.

Defining obesity presents a similar conundrum. Although humans need a certain amount of body fat to maintain basic bodily functions, excess body fat is correlated with a number of different health risks and diseases (Yach, Stuckler, & Brownell, 2006). The health consequences of obesity will be discussed in Chapters 3 and 4. The World Health Organization (WHO, 2010) defines obesity as "abnormal or excessive fat accumulation that presents a risk to health." That's all well and good, but it is not very specific. In other words, if you are trying to conduct a research study on the topic of obesity, this definition is not particularly helpful in determining who you should enroll in your study. What is "abnormal or excessive" anyway? It's sort of like saying small children shouldn't ride roller coasters. How small is too small? We need some objective cutoffs. That's where the body mass index (BMI) comes in.

By far, the most common definition of obesity uses the BMI to determine who is overweight or obese (see Table 1.1 for BMI cutoffs). A person's BMI is a ratio of his or her weight (in kilograms) to height (in meters-squared). By this metric, a BMI of 25–29.9 kg/m^2 is considered overweight and a BMI of 30 or more kg/m^2 is considered obese.

The BMI was originally called the "Quetelet index" (QI) after the Belgian mathematician who invented it (Eknoyan, 2007). Adolphe Quetelet was a mathematician and statistician

TABLE 1.1 BMI CLASSIFICATIONS
FOR ADULTS

Underweight	<18.5
Normal weight	18.5–24.99
Overweight	25–29.99
Obese	30–39.99
Extremely obese	≥40

in the 19th century who studied human growth. He discovered that weight increases as the square of height (aside from growth spurts during infancy and puberty), and subsequently created the QI, weight (in kilograms) divided by height (in meters-squared), to describe normal human growth. Approximately 100 years later (circa World War II), insurers began to report higher mortality levels among their more overweight policyholders. To account for these different levels of risk among their policyholders, actuaries started using the QI to evaluate whether policyholders were normal or overweight. Researchers thought that these insurers must be on to something and started to evaluate the QI. In the 1970s, epidemiological studies testing the validity of the QI started to emerge, and the QI was renamed BMI. Because the BMI was so easy to calculate, inexpensive, and appeared to be related to both percent body fat and morbidity and mortality risk, it was quickly adopted by researchers and health practitioners. Here we are, 40 years later, and BMI is still the most widely used metric to define and measure obesity across the globe.

You might have noticed that the BMI definition of obesity does not mention anything about body composition (i.e., bone, muscle, fat). So an NFL running back, who is 5'10" and weighs 220 lbs, would have a BMI of 31.6 kg/m^2, placing him in the obese category. However, this running back may only have a body fat percentage of 10%, hardly qualifying as obese by body fat or physical fitness standards. He is an elite athlete by one standard (percent body fat), and obese by another (BMI). On the flip side, we may have a total couch potato who is 5'6" but weighs only 130 lbs. This person has a BMI of 21 kg/m^2, perfectly healthy in terms of BMI. But with a body fat of 38%, this person may develop a number of health risks often associated with obesity.

So if we are really interested in body fat, then why do we use BMI to define obesity? It turns out that measuring body composition (e.g., percent body fat) is extremely expensive. Methods such as dual-energy x-ray absorptiometry scanning, near-infrared interactance, bioelectrical impedance analysis, and hydrostatic (underwater) weighing (just what it sounds like) can produce accurate estimates of body fat, but cost several hundred dollars or more. You need special equipment, and then people need to be trained to use the special equipment, and so on. Obviously, it is not practical to use these methods in large population studies—or even within more individualized settings, such as in a physician's office. After all, how many doctors' offices have you been to where there is a pool to do hydrostatic weighing? Even though BMI is not a perfect measure by any stretch of the imagination, it does correlate strongly with percent body fat (Flegal et al., 2009). Since BMI is so easy (and inexpensive) to calculate and it correlates so well with what we really care about (body fat), it is a pretty good proxy. Convinced? Didn't think so, but we'll talk more about that in a bit.

Defining Obesity in Kids and Adults

So you're getting ready to conduct a study looking at the prevalence of obesity among children and adults in Fiji. You have a limited budget (enough to pay for your airfare and lodging there, plus money for a scale and a tape measure). How do you determine what proportion of Fiji islanders are obese? Just look at how many people in your study sample have a BMI over 30 kg/m^2, right? Not so fast.

In adults, defining obesity is fairly straightforward. Irrespective of age, gender, race, or ethnicity, there are universal BMI cut-points that determine whether someone is underweight, normal weight, overweight, obese, or extremely obese (see Table 1.1).

In children, however, the picture gets a bit more complicated. Because children are still growing and changing, the relationship between BMI and percent body fat is not consistent. In other words, the amount of body fat in children changes with age, and it is different between boys and girls. In order to better account for this, we use something called BMI z-scores (or BMI percentiles) to determine whether children are overweight or obese (Mei et al., 2002). In addition, we have separate standards for children by age and gender (see Table 1.2). Children between the 85th and 95th percentile (for their age and gender) are considered overweight, and children who are above the 95th percentile are considered obese. You can see these growth curve trajectories in Figure 1.2.

Why Do We Use BMI Again?

As we have briefly touched upon, there are some (okay, many) drawbacks in using BMI to measure obesity. You might find the "but everyone does it that way" excuse not particularly satisfying—and you certainly wouldn't be alone. So let's discuss the pros and cons of using BMI in a little more detail.

TABLE 1.2 **BMI PERCENTILE CLASSIFICATIONS FOR CHILDREN**

Underweight	<5th percentile
Normal weight	5th–85th percentile
Overweight	85th–95th percentile
Obese	≥95th percentile

What if I'm Just Big-Boned?

Although BMI does not directly measure body fat (or muscle, or bone, for that matter), it is highly correlated with percent body fat. For men, the correlation between percent fat and BMI is between 0.72 and 0.79 (Flegal et al., 2009). For women, the

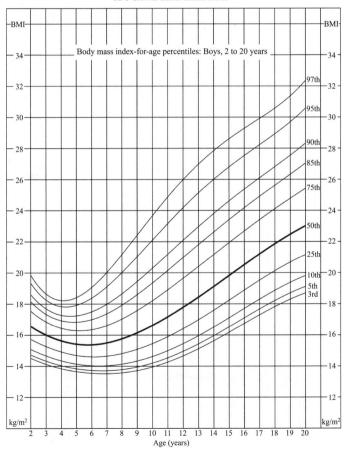

CDC Growth Charts United States

Body mass index-for-age percentiles: Boys, 2 to 20 years

FIGURE 1.2 BMI percentile charts for boys and girls. From the Centers for Disease Control and Prevention, 2009.

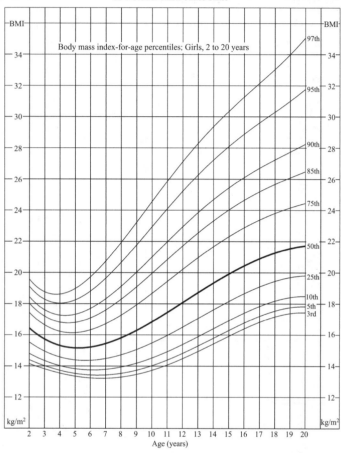

CDC Growth Charts United States

Body mass index-for-age percentiles: Girls, 2 to 20 years

FIGURE 1.2 *Continued*

correlation is between 0.72 and 0.84. (For an explanation of correlations, see Box 1.1). However, the relationship between body fat and BMI is not linear (Gallagher et al., 2000). In other words, if you go from a BMI of 22 to 23, this represents a larger change in percent body fat than if you go from a BMI of 42 to 43 (see Figure 1.3). The increases in percent body fat tend to level off at higher BMIs. It is important to note that correlations measure

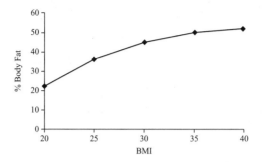

FIGURE 1.3 Relationship between BMI and percent body fat.

BOX 1.1 WHAT IS A CORRELATION?

Correlation describes how closely two things are related. Correlations (usually called *r*) range from −1 to 1. A correlation of zero indicates that two variables are completely independent or unrelated. A negative correlation means that as one variable increases, the other decreases. For example, as age increases for men, the amount of hair they have on their head decreases. This relationship or correlation is not "perfect" though because some men don't lose any hair, and some lose their hair while still young. A positive correlation means that as one variable increases, the other increases as well. For example, as height increases, weight tends to increase as well. Again, this is not a perfect correlation because some tall people are very thin and some short people are very heavy. Correlations of −1 or 1 indicate that there is a perfect, linear relationship between two variables. Importantly, correlations measure **linear** relationships. So two variables could be perfectly related, but along a curvilinear path, and the correlation may be rather low. You can see some examples in Figure 1.4.

BOX 1.1 CONTINUED

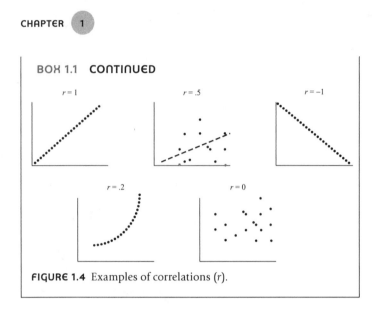

FIGURE 1.4 Examples of correlations (r).

linear relationships between two variables. So if the relationship between BMI and body fat is not linear (as we know it is not), then the correlation will be misleading (likely lower than it would be if the relationship were linear), unless adjustments are made in the analysis. Suffice it to say that the relationship between BMI and body fat is not simple.

The definition of obesity in adults is based on a cutoff of 30 kg/m^2, not a correlation value. So how well does this cutoff do in terms of identifying who has a high percent body fat? To understand this point, you need to know something about sensitivity and specificity. Sensitivity refers to how well a test identifies "true positives," and specificity refers to how well a test identifies "true negatives." Let's say we have 100 women, and we know for a fact that 25 of them are pregnant based on some fancy and tremendously expensive blood test. We want to determine the accuracy of a new (cheap) over-the-counter test, so we give it to all the women and look at the results compared with the blood test. We get Table 1.3.

In this case, the new test correctly identifies 88% of the women who are actually pregnant (sensitivity = 22/25 = 88.0%).

TABLE 1.3   AN EXAMPLE OF SENSITIVITY AND SPECIFICITY

	Definitely Pregnant	Definitely Not	
New Test Says "Pregnant"	22 (true positives)	10 (false positives)	32
New Test Says "Not"	3 (false negatives)	65 (true negatives)	68
	25	75	

It also correctly identified roughly 87% of women as not being pregnant (specificity = 65/75 = 86.6%). The new test isn't bad—but we have a handful of false positives (when the test said a woman was pregnant but she actually wasn't) and false negatives (when the test said a woman was not pregnant but, in fact, she was). So now let's apply these concepts to obesity and take a look at how well BMI does in identifying those who are obese by percent body fat standards.

Romero-Corral et al. (2008) recently looked at this issue in adults. They measured the percent body fat of participants and classified them as obese or not (more than 25% body fat is obese for men, and more than 35% body fat is obese for women). They then compared the participants' BMIs to their body fat. First, the good news. BMI does a very good job at correctly identifying true negatives. That is, the specificity of BMI is high—95% for men and 99% for women. This means that for men and women who have low body fat percentages, they are also likely to fall into the normal weight range by BMI standards. Now the bad news. The sensitivity of BMI is pretty terrible—36% for men and 49% for women. This means that a BMI of 30 kg/m^2 catches less than half (!) of those men and women who would be considered obese based on their percent body fat. In other words, there are a lot of people with high percent body fat who have normal BMIs.

In children, BMI percentile cutoffs perform better than BMI cutoffs in adults. First, recall that obesity in children is defined as having a higher BMI than 95% of children in a reference group of the same age and gender. Using this metric, the sensitivity of BMI cutoffs in children is 70% to 80%, and the specificity is 95% (Freeman & Sherry, 2009). So the age- and gender-specific cutoffs for children correctly identify about three out of four obese children, and correctly classify nearly all of the nonobese children.

Many times BMI is criticized for the false positives, where very muscular people are deemed to be obese despite ultralow body fat levels. However, very high specificities indicate that this happens pretty infrequently. A *much* larger problem is the issue of false negatives, where people who are actually obese by percent body fat standards are not captured by just looking at their BMI. If we were looking at cases of cancer, for example, what would you consider to be a larger concern: (a) a handful of individuals who are incorrectly diagnosed as having cancer when they do not or (b) the fact that more than half of individuals who actually have cancer are incorrectly told that they are healthy? Obviously, there are differences between obesity and cancer that would lead us to accept different thresholds for measurement errors, but it is an interesting point to think about.

A second important consequence of this measurement error is the effect on studies of the relationships between obesity and various diseases. We will spare you the statistical details and skip right to the take-home point: measurement error is very bad for your research. Let's say you want to look at the relationship between kids' candy intake and hyperactivity. To measure these things, you ask 4-year-old children how often they eat candy, and then you ask them "do you feel hyper?" Are you likely to get an accurate picture of candy intake and hyperactivity from these questions? Probably not. Kids may say they eat less candy than they do because their mom is in the room, or maybe they had a piece of candy yesterday so they respond "a lot" even though they rarely have candy. Similarly, do you trust a 4-year-old's self-report of hyperactivity? You might as well flip a coin (heads means hyper, tails means not). Clearly, there is a lot of measurement error in this scenario—it's not exactly clear what you are even measuring, but it's probably not very closely related to actual candy intake or hyperactivity. So when you go to do your analysis looking at the relationship between these two variables, you aren't likely to find anything meaningful (even if there is, in fact, a very strong relationship between the two variables). Looking at how this might apply to studies of obesity, we can see that using BMI to define and measure obesity may pose a problem for research looking at relationships between obesity and a variety of outcomes. This point will be relevant when we talk about the consequences of obesity in subsequent chapters.

Getting back to some other criticisms of BMI, you might have noticed that Romero-Corral et al. (2008) tested men and women separately. This brings up another criticism of BMI, in that we use the same formula and the same cutoffs for all men and women, regardless of their gender, age, race, or ethnicity. We know that men and women have different levels of muscle mass and body fat, so why would we use the same metric to determine whether or not they are obese? We use age- and gender-adjusted formulas for calculating BMI z-score or percentile in children, so why do we use a "one-size-fits-all" approach for adults? Again, the very unsatisfying answer is "it's simpler to have one metric" and, historically, that's just the way everyone does it.

The relationship between BMI and body fat not only differs between men and women but also differs by age and between different racial and ethnic groups (Flegal et al., 2009; Gallagher et al., 2000; Sumner, Ricks, Sen, & Frempong, 2007). You can see this in Table 1.4. Moreover, BMI relates differently to health risks in different age groups and different racial and ethnic groups (Sumner et al., 2007). For example, South Asian people tend to have a higher percent body fat than Caucasian people at all BMI levels, and this higher percent body fat likely puts South

TABLE 1.4 PERCENT BODY FAT CORRESPONDING TO BMI CUT-POINTS BY AGE, RACE/ETHNICITY, AND GENDER

	Women			Men		
	African American (%)	Asian (%)	Caucasian (%)	African American (%)	Asian (%)	Caucasian (%)
20–39 years						
BMI < 18.5	20	25	21	8	13	8
BMI > 25	32	35	33	20	23	21
BMI > 30	38	40	39	26	28	26
40–59 years						
BMI < 18.5	21	25	23	9	13	11
BMI > 25	34	36	35	22	24	23
BMI > 30	39	41	41	27	29	29
60–79 years						
BMI < 18.5	23	26	25	11	14	13
BMI > 25	35	36	38	23	24	25
BMI > 30	41	41	43	29	29	31

From Sumner et al., 2007.

Asian people at risk for negative health outcomes (e.g., diabetes, heart disease) at lower BMIs than we typically see in Caucasian people (Sumner et al., 2007).

Are There Other Measures of Obesity?

In a word, yes. There are plenty of other measures. You could measure body composition (e.g., percent body fat, percent muscle mass) using some of the techniques we already listed, but these are expensive. In addition, there are other measures such as waist circumference or waist-to-hip ratio (WHR) that correlate with body fat. In fact, waist circumference correlates more closely with body fat among men, but BMI correlates better with body fat among women (Flegal et al., 2009). Waist circumference or WHR measures something called "abdominal or central obesity," a condition that is closely related to negative health outcomes such as cardiovascular disease (de Koning, Merchant, Pogue, & Anand, 2007). It is not just how much body fat you have that relates to your health, but where that body fat is located. People who are apple shaped tend to have worse health outcomes than people who are pear shaped (Hamdy, Porramatikul, & Al-Ozairi, 2006). For those who don't visit the produce section on a regular basis, high concentrations of body fat around the midsection, notably the abdominal area, are associated with worse health outcomes than if body fat is more evenly distributed or more concentrated in the lower body, for example.

Again, we are back to the question, "Why do we use BMI?" There seem to be a lot of limitations to this metric. This really boils down to the fact that BMI was developed in the 1800s to assess normal human growth. The research needs of today may not be well served by metrics devised 200 years ago; nothing personal against the 19th century. Moreover, BMI was co-opted by researchers after it rose in popularity due to its utility to insurers for calculating which policyholders to charge higher premiums. Research is now beginning to incorporate alternative measures of adiposity (e.g., waist circumferences or WHRs) to at least supplement BMI in studies of obesity. Researchers with lots of funding are able to use more expensive and superior measures of body composition. However, despite all of the known drawbacks to using BMI to define and measure obesity, it is unlikely that we will see a shift in this metric's popularity any time soon. Because it is used so pervasively and is so easy and inexpensive to calculate, BMI will continue to be the most commonly used metric to define and measure obesity in both research and practice for many years to come.

Fully admitting we are part of the problem, we will use the BMI-based definition of obesity throughout the rest of this book (unless otherwise specified).

WHY SHOULD WE CARE ABOUT OBESITY?

The bottom line is that obesity is bad for your health. We will talk about this in much greater detail in subsequent chapters, but suffice it to say obesity is related to dozens of negative outcomes, including:

- Hypertension or high blood pressure (Brown et al., 2000; Mokdad et al., 2003)
- Dyslipidemia or high cholesterol and triglycerides (Brown et al., 2000)
- Type 2 diabetes (National Task Force on the Prevention and Treatment of Obesity, 2000)
- Coronary heart or cardiovascular disease (Gregg et al., 2005)
- Stroke (Cooper et al., 2000; Strazzullo et al., 2010)
- Osteoarthritis and musculoskeletal problems (Anandacoomarasamy, Fransen, & March, 2009)
- Sleep apnea and other respiratory problems (de Sousa, Cercato, Mancini, & Halpern, 2008)

- Endometrial, breast, prostate, pancreatic, esophageal, kidney, liver, gallbladder, and colon cancers (Percik & Stumvoll, 2009; Pischon, Nothlings, & Boeing, 2008; Renehan, Tyson, Egger, Heller, & Zwahlen, 2008)
- Depression, anxiety, and lower quality of life (Fontaine & Barofsky, 2001; Luppino et al., 2010; Wadden, Womble, Stunkard, & Anderson, 2002)
- Frailty in older adults (Blaum, Xue, Michelon, Semba, & Fried, 2005)
- Dementia (Beydoun, Beydoun, & Wang, 2008)
- Reductions in life expectancy (Fontaine, Redden, Wang, Westfall, & Allison, 2003; Peeters et al., 2003; St. Onge & Heymsfield, 2003)
- Mortality (Flegal, Graubard, Williamson, & Gail, 2005, 2007; Mokdad, Marks, Stroup, & Gerberding, 2004)

As obesity becomes much more common, so do these negative health consequences. This is a concern not only for the vast number of individuals who now have to deal with these health issues but also for society at large. The costs to society of obesity and related health issues are tremendous.

PREVALENCE OF OBESITY IN THE UNITED STATES

Obesity Among Adults

If you have been to a beach lately, or a sports game, or Disney World, or a concert, or a restaurant, or the movies, or have walked down a crowded street...or been basically any place where there are large numbers of people, then you probably couldn't help but notice that obesity is extremely common. More than two thirds of Americans are now overweight or obese (68% have a BMI over 25 kg/m^2; Flegal, Carroll, Ogden, & Curtin, 2010), meaning that less than one third of American adults are of a healthy weight. These estimates of prevalence come from a national survey conducted every few years by the National Health and Nutrition Examination Survey (NHANES; Centers for Disease Control and Prevention, 2010a). This survey actually measures participants' heights and weights (and a variety of other things), in contrast to many other surveys and studies that rely on self-reported height and weight. This is important for estimating prevalence because when people report their own height and weight, they tend to overstate their height and understate their weight (who wouldn't shave off a few pounds when asked?). So NHANES is really considered the gold standard for assessing the prevalence of obesity in the United States.

We would be remiss if we did not mention another national survey conducted each year by the Centers for Disease Control and Prevention (CDC), the Behavioral Risk Factor Surveillance Survey (BRFSS; Centers for Disease Control and Prevention, 2010b). This survey is conducted by phone, so it relies on self-reported heights and weights, which tend to underestimate obesity levels. However, the BRFSS is very useful for two reasons. First, we can see trends over time. The CDC has created a very cool map illustrating the increasing prevalence of obesity over time in the United States.[1] Although these prevalence estimates are artificially low, it does demonstrate that obesity has become much more common over the past 20 years. Second, the sample of people surveyed in the BRFSS is representative at the county level. The NHANES looks at a nationally representative sample, so we cannot look at individual states or compare counties using the NHANES. When we want to look at state- or county-level estimates of obesity prevalence (e.g., if we want to look at whether obesity is more prevalent in urban or rural counties, or in the south versus the northeast), we have to rely on the BRFSS.

Any way you gather or slice the data, it is clear that prior to the 1960s, obesity was not considered to be the threat to public health that it is today. The prevalence of obesity among

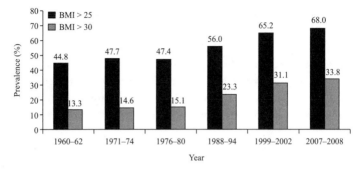

FIGURE 1.5 Prevalence of obesity and overweight among adults by year in the United States.

American adults in 1960 to 1962 was only 13.4% (Flegal, Carroll, Ogden, & Johnson, 2002). Fast forward to present day, and the prevalence of obesity among U.S. adults is now 33.8% (Flegal et al., 2010). You can see these changes in prevalence of obesity over time in Figure 1.5.

Sometimes, these numbers can get confusing, because some percentages include only obese individuals and some include both overweight and obese individuals. To clarify and summarize the take-home point here, the most recent estimates suggest that about one third of American adults are obese and another one third are overweight. This means that more than two thirds of American adults are *either* overweight or obese. With a few seconds of basic math, you realize that being "normal" weight is no longer the norm—fewer than one in three American adults is of a "normal" or healthy weight.

Obesity Among Children

Twenty years ago, you probably could have gotten through an entire month or even year without hearing about childhood obesity. Now, it seems the topic is constantly in the media, being discussed everywhere from TV talk shows and news to your latest PTA meeting. If you have kids, maybe your pediatrician has even broached the topic. Or perhaps you have heard other adults reminiscing about how they used to play on the streets as children, whereas kids now stay inside playing video games. What is clear is that discussions of childhood obesity are now ubiquitous. This is for good reason; while a smaller proportion of children are overweight or obese as compared with adults, the prevalence of obesity among children in the United States has grown even more rapidly over the past few decades than we have seen for adults.

Estimates from NHANES indicate that in the early 1970s, the prevalence of obesity among children was between 4.0% and 6.1% (Centers for Disease Control and Prevention, 2010c). Fast forward again to between 2003 and 2006, and we see that between 30.1% and 33.6% of children in the United States were overweight or obese (BMI at or above the 85th percentile for age and gender) and 12.4% to 17.6% are obese (at or above the 95th percentile for age and gender; Ogden, Carroll, & Curtin, 2006; Ogden, Carroll, & Flegal, 2008). The most recent estimates suggest that 31.7% of children were overweight or obese, and 16.9% were obese in 2007 to 2008 (Ogden, Carroll, Curtin, Lamb, & Flegal, 2010). Perhaps the most alarming statistic is that the percentage of children who are obese has grown by

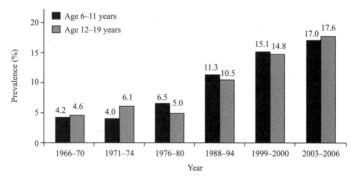

FIGURE 1.6 Prevalence of obesity among children by year in the United States.

approximately 400% over the past 4 decades. You can see these changes over time in Figure 1.6.

DISPARITIES

While the obesity epidemic has impacted virtually all segments of the population, certain subgroups are disproportionately affected. Women, ethnic and racial subgroups, and those of low socioeconomic status (SES) all display higher rates of obesity than the overall population (Flegal et al., 2002, 2010; Hedley et al., 2004).

Racial/Ethnic Differences

Obesity is much more common in certain racial and ethnic subpopulations, as compared with Caucasian Americans. For example, 44.1% of non-Hispanic African Americans, 38.7% of Hispanic Americans, and 40.4% of Mexican Americans are obese (Flegal et al., 2010). These percentages are higher than the 32.4% of obese non-Hispanic Caucasian Americans (Flegal et al., 2010). Among children as well, obesity is more prevalent in some racial and ethnic subpopulations (i.e., Mexican American and non-Hispanic African American children; Ogden et al., 2010; Wang & Beydoun, 2007).

Several reasons have been proposed to account for these disparities. It has been suggested that there are cultural differences in eating patterns and body image between certain racial and ethnic subgroups (Kumanyika, 2008). It has also been suggested that these differences are really driven by socioeconomic disparities, and because race and ethnicity and income are so intertwined, you cannot tease apart the effects of either (Kumanyika, 2008). Finally, some have suggested that these differences reflect different environments in which racial and ethnic subpopulations tend to live (Kumanyika, 2008;

Yancey & Kumanyika, 2007). For example, predominantly African American or low-income neighborhoods are more likely to have a fast food restaurant nearby, and be further away from a grocery store, than predominantly Caucasian American or higher income neighborhoods (Gordon-Larsen, Nelson, Page, & Popkin, 2006; Story, Kaphingst, Robinson-O'Brien, & Glanz, 2008; Yancey & Kumanyika, 2007). This topic will be discussed in detail later in the book.

Gender Differences

In general, women are more likely to be obese than men (see Figure 1.7). The prevalence of obesity among women is 35.5% compared with 32.2% for men (Flegal et al., 2010). Some of the most startling estimates of obesity prevalence are among subgroups of women. For example, almost half (49.6%) of non-Hispanic African American women are obese (Flegal et al., 2010).

Socioeconomic Differences

Income is related to obesity, though this relationship is not uniform across the globe. In the United States (and other

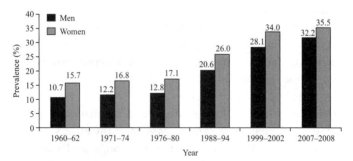

FIGURE 1.7 Prevalence of obesity among men and women by year in the United States.

developed nations), people living in poverty are more likely to be obese than those with higher incomes (Baum & Ruhm, 2009; Runge, 2007; Sturm, 2008). Education is also related to obesity. Those with higher levels of education are less likely to be obese than individuals with less education (Sturm, 2008). Overweight or obesity is more prevalent in children whose parents are of low education or low income (Wang, 2001; Wang & Beydoun, 2007). However, these socioeconomic differences have become narrower over the past several decades, suggesting that individual-level factors, such as education, are less important than the broader socioeconomic and environmental contexts in which people live (Zhang & Wang, 2004).

Many possible explanations have been proposed for SES disparities in obesity, similar to racial and ethnic disparities. Some have suggested that higher levels of education mean that individuals have greater knowledge about health and health behaviors, which has been referred to as "health literacy" (Sanders, Shaw, Guez, Baur, & Rudd, 2009). Some have suggested that SES differences are due to the fact that lower-income people cannot afford to eat healthier foods, such as whole grains and fresh fruits and vegetables, because these foods are more expensive than convenience or fast food items (Drewnowski & Specter, 2004). If you have ever attempted to buy a meal at Whole Foods, this probably comes as no surprise. Hitting up the Burger King drive-through will save you a substantial amount of money by comparison. Some have suggested that SES differences are driven by the different environments that low-income people live in compared with higher-income people. For example, low-income neighborhoods have fewer supermarkets and more convenience stores and fast food restaurants (Gordon-Larsen et al., 2006; Story et al., 2008). There are many other environmental factors that may predispose low-income individuals to obesity. We will discuss these factors in much greater detail later on in the book. Finally, obesity is associated with lower-paying jobs or lower wages, which further limits the ability to afford a healthy diet or an expensive gym membership. We will discuss occupational outcomes for overweight and obese individuals in Chapter 3.

At this point, you can see that the relationships tying income, education, gender, race, and ethnicity to obesity are complex, and cannot be boiled down to a simple X causes Y pathway. We will discuss these and many other factors in later chapters where we talk about the causes of obesity.

ECONOMIC IMPACTS OF OBESITY

Hopefully, we have begun to convince you that obesity is a problem worth looking at because of the effects it has on our health (if not, we'll keep trying in later chapters, don't worry). However, maybe you are one of those naturally thin people out there who says, "sure, it stinks for those people who are obese, but it's not my problem." Well, actually, even if you don't fall into the overweight or obese category and are otherwise perfectly healthy, obesity may be your problem too, or at least your wallet's problem. Obesity and related health conditions cost us a lot of money—all of us, regardless of our own weight, age, or health status.

Individual Level

Obviously, individuals who are obese face greater personal costs in terms of health care. They are more likely to have a host of other health conditions that lead to increased medical care and prescription drug use. Obese individuals pay almost $1,500 more each year on health care than normal weight individuals (Finkelstein, Trogdon, Cohen, & Dietz, 2009). Weight-loss treatment is often not covered by insurance, so overweight and obese people typically have to pay out of pocket for these services that may include anything from nutritional counseling to surgery (in addition to various over-the-counter or commercial weight-loss programs that obese individuals may use).

There may also be some costs for obese individuals that you may not have thought about, such as lower wages because of work-place discrimination (Cawley, 2004, 2010), higher gasoline costs (because it requires more gas to transport heavier cars and planes), more expensive clothing or tailoring, or having to buy two seats on an airplane (Jacobson & McLay, 2006; McCormick, Stone, & Corporate Analytical Team, 2007). All in all, it is not only bad for your health to be obese but also bad for your personal finances.

Societal or Government Level

The costs of obesity are high not only for obese individuals but also for society at large and for our government (or us, as taxpayers). Whereas an obese person may have to buy two airline tickets, we all pay more for tickets regardless of our weights (because more obese passengers means higher fuel costs for the airlines; Jacobson & Mclay, 2006; McCormick, Stone, & Corporate Analytical Team, 2007). More concerning is the tremendous costs of health care related to obesity. Approximately 10% of the nation's health care expenditures are related to obesity (Finkelstein, Fiebelkorn, & Wang, 2003; Ludwig & Pollack, 2009). Treating obesity and related illnesses costs $147 billion each year in the United States (Cawley, 2010; Finkelstein et al., 2009). These costs *only* include those related to health care, and does not include missed workdays or lost productivity due to obesity and related diseases. Some have suggested the actual direct costs may be twice this amount when you include other factors besides health care costs (Ludwig & Pollack, 2009).

If you have private health insurance, you likely pay a higher premium because the prevalence of obesity and related health care costs has increased so drastically. Health care costs for obese individuals are 37% higher than those for normal weight individuals (Finkelstein et al., 2003; Loureiro, 2004). Unless your insurance company charges you according to your weight, these costs are spread out over the entire pool of insured people, including those who are healthy and thin. What this means is that we all pay an extra $732 for health care, regardless of our own weight or health status (Finkelstein et al., 2003; Loureiro, 2004).

Because our employers typically pay a portion of our health insurance premiums, the costs due to obesity affect employers as well. Cost claims are twice as high for obese children and adults than normal-weight children and adults (Sepulveda, Tait, Zimmerman, & Edington, 2010). Employers also face the costs related to lost productivity and missed work. Obesity and related health issues result in $4.3 billion in lost workdays each year and $506 lost per obese worker due to lower productivity while at work (Cawley, 2010; Cawley, Rizzo, & Haas, 2007; Gates, Succop, Brehm, Gillespie, & Sommers, 2008).

Governments are faced with increased costs related to Medicare and Medicaid, Veteran's health care, disability programs, and workforce productivity issues (e.g., obesity in the military). These costs are borne by the taxpayers (i.e., we the people). In 2008, obesity-related illnesses cost Medicare and Medicaid $27.7 billion (Cawley, 2010; Finkelstein et al., 2009), an amount that we all pay for in the form of taxes.

PREVIEW OF WHAT'S TO COME

Now that you know what exactly obesity is, how it is measured, and why we should care about it, we will move on to discuss what causes it. Is it our genes? Is it an evil conspiracy on the part of McDonald's and Burger King? Is it our environment? Is it food advertising? Is it our parents? None of the above? All of the above?

We will then discuss the numerous medical and psychosocial consequences of obesity in much greater detail. In Chapter 5, we will discuss various treatments for obesity, and how effective they are. In Chapter 6, we will discuss the prevention of obesity. Finally, we will wrap up with a discussion of future trends and global issues related to obesity.

NOTE

[1]You can see this map at http://www.cdc.gov/obesity/data/trends.html#State

REFERENCES

Anandacoomarasamy, A., Fransen, M., & March, L. (2009). Obesity and the musculoskeletal system. *Current Opinion in Rheumatology*, *21*(1), 71–77.

Baum, C. L., & Ruhm, C. J. (2009). Age, socioeconomic status and obesity growth. *Journal of Health Economics*, *28*(3), 635–648.

Beydoun, M. A., Beydoun, H. A., & Wang, Y. (2008). Obesity and central obesity as risk factors for incident dementia and its subtypes: A systematic review and meta-analysis. *Obesity Reviews: An Official Journal of the International Association for the Study of Obesity*, *9*(3), 204–218.

Blaum, C. S., Xue, Q. L., Michelon, E., Semba, R. D., & Fried, L. P. (2005). The association between obesity and the frailty syndrome in older women: The Women's Health and Aging Studies. *Journal of the American Geriatrics Society*, *53*(6), 927–934.

Brown, C. D., Higgins, M., Donato, K. A., Rohde, F. C., Garrison, R., Obarzanek, E.,...Horan, M. (2000). Body mass index and the prevalence of hypertension and dyslipidemia. *Obesity Research*, *8*(9), 605–619.

Cawley, J. (2004). The impact of obesity on wages. *Journal of Human Resources*, *39*, 451–474.

Cawley, J. (2010). The economics of childhood obesity. *Health Affairs (Project Hope)*, *29*(3), 364–371.

Cawley, J., Rizzo, J. A., & Haas, K. (2007). Occupation-specific absenteeism costs associated with obesity and morbid obesity. *Journal of Occupational and Environmental Medicine/American College of Occupational and Environmental Medicine, 49*(12), 1317–1324.

Centers for Disease Control and Prevention. (2009). *Clinical Growth Charts.* Retrieved February 22, 2011, from http://www.cdc.gov/growthcharts/clinical_charts.htm

Centers for Disease Control and Prevention. (2010a). *National Health and Nutrition Examination Survey.* Retrieved February 16, 2011, from http://www.cdc.gov/nhanes

Centers for Disease Control and Prevention. (2010b). *Behavioral Risk Factor Surveillance System* (BRFSS). Retrieved February 16, 2011, from http://www.cdc.gov/BRFSS

Centers for Disease Control and Prevention. (2010c). *U.S. Obesity Trends.* Retrieved February 16, 2011, from http://www.cdc.gov/obesity/data/trends.html

Cooper, R., Cutler, J., Desvigne-Nickens, P., Fortmann, S. P., Friedman, L., Havlik, R.,...Thom, T. (2000). Trends and disparities in coronary heart disease, stroke, and other cardiovascular diseases in the United States: Findings of the national conference on cardiovascular disease prevention. *Circulation, 102*(25), 3137–3147.

de Koning, L., Merchant, A. T., Pogue, J., & Anand, S. S. (2007). Waist circumference and waist-to-hip ratio as predictors of cardiovascular events: Meta-regression analysis of prospective studies. *European Heart Journal, 28*(7), 850–856.

de Sousa, A. G., Cercato, C., Mancini, M. C., & Halpern, A. (2008). Obesity and obstructive sleep apnea-hypopnea syndrome. *Obesity Reviews: An Official Journal of the International Association for the Study of Obesity, 9*(4), 340–354.

Drewnowski, A., & Specter, S. E. (2004). Poverty and obesity: The role of energy density and energy costs. *American Journal of Clinical Nutrition, 79*(1), 6–16.

Eknoyan, G. (2008). Adolphe Quetelet (1796–1874)—The average man and indices of obesity. *Nephrology, Dialysis, Transplantation: Official Publication of the European Dialysis and Transplant Association—European Renal Association, 23*(1), 47–51.

Finkelstein, E. A., Fiebelkorn, I. C., & Wang, G. (2003). National medical spending attributable to overweight and obesity: How much, and who's paying? *Health Affairs (Project Hope), Suppl Web Exclusives*, W3–219.

Finkelstein, E. A., Trogdon, J. G., Cohen, J. W., & Dietz, W. (2009). Annual medical spending attributable to obesity: Payer- and service-specific estimates. *Health Affairs (Project Hope)*, *28*(5), w822–w831.

Flegal, K. M., Carroll, M. D., Ogden, C. L., & Curtin, L. R. (2010). Prevalence and trends in obesity among US adults, 1999–2008. *The Journal of the American Medical Association*, *303*(3), 235–241.

Flegal, K. M., Carroll, M. D., Ogden, C. L., & Johnson, C. L. (2002). Prevalence and trends in obesity among US adults, 1999–2000. *The Journal of the American Medical Association*, *288*(14), 1723–1727.

Flegal, K. M., Graubard, B. I., Williamson, D. F., & Gail, M. H. (2005). Excess deaths associated with underweight, overweight, and obesity. *The Journal of the American Medical Association*, *293*(15), 1861–1867.

Flegal, K. M., Graubard, B. I., Williamson, D. F., & Gail, M. H. (2007). Cause-specific excess deaths associated with underweight, overweight, and obesity. *The Journal of the American Medical Association*, *298*(17), 2028–2037.

Flegal, K. M., Shepherd, J. A., Looker, A. C., Graubard, B. I., Borrud, L. G., Ogden, C. L.,…Schenker, N. (2009). Comparisons of percentage body fat, body mass index, waist circumference, and waist-stature ratio in adults. *American Journal of Clinical Nutrition*, *89*(2), 500–508.

Fontaine, K. R., & Barofsky, I. (2001). Obesity and health-related quality of life. *Obesity Reviews: An Official Journal of the International Association for the Study of Obesity*, *2*(3), 173–182.

Fontaine, K. R., Redden, D. T., Wang, C., Westfall, A. O., & Allison, D. B. (2003). Years of life lost due to obesity. *The Journal of the American Medical Association*, *289*(2), 187–193.

Freedman, D. S., & Sherry, B. (2009). The validity of BMI as an indicator of body fatness and risk among children. *Pediatrics*, *124*(Suppl. 1), S23–S34.

Gallagher, D., Heymsfield, S. B., Heo, M., Jebb, S. A., Murgatroyd, P. R., & Sakamoto, Y. (2000). Healthy percentage body fat ranges: An approach for developing guidelines based on body mass index. *American Journal of Clinical Nutrition*, *72*(3), 694–701.

Gates, D. M., Succop, P., Brehm, B. J., Gillespie, G. L., & Sommers, B. D. (2008). Obesity and presenteeism: The impact of body mass index on workplace productivity. *Journal of Occupational and Environmental Medicine/American College of Occupational and Environmental Medicine, 50*(1), 39–45.

Gordon-Larsen, P., Nelson, M. C., Page, P., & Popkin, B. M. (2006). Inequality in the built environment underlies key health disparities in physical activity and obesity. *Pediatrics, 117*(2), 417–424.

Gregg, E. W., Cheng, Y. J., Cadwell, B. L., Imperatore, G., Williams, D. E., Flegal, K. M.,...Williamson, D. F. (2005). Secular trends in cardiovascular disease risk factors according to body mass index in US adults. *The Journal of the American Medical Association, 293*(15), 1868–1874.

Hamdy, O., Porramatikul, S., & Al-Ozairi, E. (2006). Metabolic obesity: The paradox between visceral and subcutaneous fat. *Current Diabetes Reviews, 2*(4), 367–373.

Hedley, A. A., Ogden, C. L., Johnson, C. L., Carroll, M. D., Curtin, L. R., & Flegal, K. M. (2004). Prevalence of overweight and obesity among US children, adolescents, and adults, 1999–2002. *The Journal of the American Medical Association, 291*(23), 2847–2850.

Jacobson, S. H., & McLay, L. A. (2006). The economic impact of obesity on automobile fuel consumption. *The Engineering Economist, 51*(4), 307–323.

Kumanyika, S. K. (2008). Environmental influences on childhood obesity: Ethnic and cultural influences in context. *Physiology & Behavior, 94*(1), 61–70.

Loureiro, M. L. (2004). Obesity: Economic dimensions of a 'super size' problem. *Choices, 19*(3), 35–39.

Ludwig, D. S., & Pollack, H. A. (2009). Obesity and the economy: From crisis to opportunity. *The Journal of the American Medical Association, 301*(5), 533–535.

Luppino, F. S., de Wit, L. M., Bouvy, P. F., Stijnen, T., Cuijpers, P., Penninx, B. W., & Zitman, F. G. (2010). Overweight, obesity, and depression: A systematic review and meta-analysis of longitudinal studies. *Archives of General Psychiatry, 67*(3), 220–229.

McCormick, B., Stone, I., & Corporate Analytical Team. (2007). Economic costs of obesity and the case for government intervention. *Obesity Reviews: An Official Journal of the International Association for the Study of Obesity, 8*(Suppl. 1), 161–164.

Mei, Z., Grummer-Strawn, L. M., Pietrobelli, A., Goulding, A., Goran, M. I., & Dietz, W. H. (2002). Validity of body mass index compared with other body-composition screening indexes for the assessment of body fatness in children and adolescents. *American Journal of Clinical Nutrition, 75*(6), 978–985.

Mokdad, A. H., Ford, E. S., Bowman, B. A., Dietz, W. H., Vinicor, F., Bales, V. S., & Marks, J. S. (2003). Prevalence of obesity, diabetes, and obesity-related health risk factors, 2001. *The Journal of the American Medical Association, 289*(1), 76–79.

Mokdad, A. H., Marks, J. S., Stroup, D. F., & Gerberding, J. L. (2004). Actual causes of death in the United States, 2000. *The Journal of the American Medical Association, 291*(10), 1238–1245.

National Task Force on the Prevention and Treatment of Obesity. (2000). Overweight, obesity, and health risk. *Archives of Internal Medicine, 160*, 898–904.

Ogden, C. L., Carroll, M. D., Curtin, L. R., Lamb, M. M., & Flegal, K. M. (2010). Prevalence of high body mass index in US children and adolescents, 2007–2008. *The Journal of the American Medical Association, 303*(3), 242–249.

Ogden, C. L., Carroll, M. D., Curtin, L. R., McDowell, M. A., Tabak, C. J., & Flegal, K. M. (2006). Prevalence of overweight and obesity in the United States, 1999–2004. *The Journal of the American Medical Association, 295*(13), 1549–1555.

Ogden, C. L., Carroll, M. D., & Flegal, K. M. (2008). High body mass index for age among US children and adolescents, 2003–2006. *The Journal of the American Medical Association, 299*(20), 2401–2405.

Peeters, A., Barendregt, J. J., Willekens, F., Mackenbach, J. P., Al Mamun, A., & Bonneux, L.; NEDCOM, the Netherlands Epidemiology and Demography Compression of Morbidity Research Group. (2003). Obesity in adulthood and its consequences for life expectancy: A life-table analysis. *Annals of Internal Medicine, 138*(1), 24–32.

Percik, R., & Stumvoll, M. (2009). Obesity and cancer. *Experimental and Clinical Endocrinology & Diabetes: Official Journal, German Society of Endocrinology [and] German Diabetes Association, 117*(10), 563–566.

Pischon, T., Nöthlings, U., & Boeing, H. (2008). Obesity and cancer. *The Proceedings of the Nutrition Society, 67*(2), 128–145.

Renehan, A. G., Tyson, M., Egger, M., Heller, R. F., & Zwahlen, M. (2008). Body-mass index and incidence of cancer: A systematic review and meta-analysis of prospective observational studies. *Lancet, 371*(9612), 569–578.

Romero-Corral, A., Somers, V. K., Sierra-Johnson, J., Thomas, R. J., Collazo-Clavell, M. L., Korinek, J.,...Lopez-Jimenez, F. (2008). Accuracy of body mass index in diagnosing obesity in the adult general population. *International Journal of Obesity*, *32*(6), 959–966.

Runge, C. F. (2007). Economic consequences of the obese. *Diabetes*, *56*(11), 2668–2672.

Sanders, L. M., Shaw, J. S., Guez, G., Baur, C., & Rudd, R. (2009). Health literacy and child health promotion: Implications for research, clinical care, and public policy. *Pediatrics*, *124*(Suppl. 3), S306–S314.

Sepulveda, M. J., Tait, F., Zimmerman, E., & Edington, D. (2010). Impact of childhood obesity on employers. *Health Affairs (Project Hope)*, *29*(3), 513–521.

St. Onge, M. P., & Heymsfield, S. B. (2003). Overweight and obesity status are linked to lower life expectancy. *Nutrition Reviews*, *61*(9), 313–316.

Story, M., Kaphingst, K. M., Robinson-O'Brien, R., & Glanz, K. (2008). Creating healthy food and eating environments: Policy and environmental approaches. *Annual Review of Public Health*, *29*, 253–272.

Strazzullo, P., D'Elia, L., Cairella, G., Garbagnati, F., Cappuccio, F. P., & Scalfi, L. (2010). Excess body weight and incidence of stroke: Meta-analysis of prospective studies with 2 million participants. *Stroke; a Journal of Cerebral Circulation*, *41*(5), e418–e426.

Sturm, R. (2008). Stemming the global obesity epidemic: What can we learn from data about social and economic trends? *Public Health*, *122*(8), 739–746.

Sumner, A. E., Ricks, M., Sen, S., & Frempong, B. A. (2007). How current guidelines for obesity underestimate risk in certain ethnicities and overestimate risk in others. *Current Cardiovascular Risk Reports*, *1*(2), 97–101.

Wadden, T. A., Womble, L. G., Stunkard, A. J., & Anderson, D. A. (2002). Psychosocial consequences of obesity and weight loss. In T. A. Wadden & A. J. Stunkard (Eds.), *Handbook of obesity treatment* (pp. 144–169). New York: Guilford Press.

Wang, Y. (2001). Cross-national comparison of childhood obesity: The epidemic and the relationship between obesity and socioeconomic status. *International Journal of Epidemiology*, *30*(5), 1129–1136.

Wang, Y., & Beydoun, M. A. (2007). The obesity epidemic in the United States–gender, age, socioeconomic, racial/ethnic, and geographic characteristics: A systematic review and meta-regression analysis. *Epidemiologic Reviews, 29,* 6–28.

World Health Organization. (2010). *Obesity.* Retrieved February 16, 2011, from http://www.who.int/topics/obesity/en/

Yach, D., Stuckler, D., & Brownell, K. D. (2006). Epidemiologic and economic consequences of the global epidemics of obesity and diabetes. *Nature Medicine, 12*(1), 62–66.

Yancey, A. K., & Kumanyika, S. K. (2007). Bridging the Gap: Understanding the structure of social inequities in childhood obesity. *American Journal of Preventive Medicine, 33*(4 Suppl.), S172–S174.

Zhang, Q., & Wang, Y. (2004). Trends in the association between obesity and socioeconomic status in U.S. adults: 1971 to 2000. *Obesity Research, 12*(10), 1622–1632.

Causes of Obesity

There are enough theories out there regarding what causes obesity to make your head spin. Here are a few cited causes (in no particular order) to help give you an idea of the various factors that have been linked to obesity: lack of sleep, what mom eats when you are in the womb, a few hundred different genes, hormones, several medical conditions, some medicines, fast food, soda, video games, pollution, air conditioning, TV, stress, depression, poverty, age, pregnancy, marriage, certain viruses, bacteria in the gut, skipping breakfast, quitting smoking, food advertising, too much sugar, too much fat, too many carbohydrates, too much snacking, food addictions, and the list goes on, and on, and on. We will discuss all of these (and more!) in this chapter. Buckle your seatbelts.

ΠATURE VS. ΠURTURE...
IT'S ALL MOM AND DAD'S FAULT, RIGHT?

Over the course of several years, we have had hundreds of conversations about obesity with friends, relatives, and complete strangers. The vast majority of these conversations have centered on what causes obesity, and what accounts for the continued increases in the prevalence of obesity. For some reason, this seems to be a topic that generates tremendous interest, curiosity, and some very strong opinions. Even people who have never read a paper on obesity seem to have an opinion about what causes it (and usually they voice these opinions very loudly and confidently). In our experience, these opinions generally fall into one of two camps: the nature camp or the nurture camp.

The nature camp believes that obesity is genetic—that as soon as the sperm fertilizes that egg, we are fated to a certain body weight purely by virtue of our DNA. This view can be oddly comforting to people who hate to diet. After all, what's the point of dieting if your genes command your body to maintain a certain weight? It also makes intuitive sense. If physical characteristics such as our (real) hair color, eye color, height, and shoe size are determined by our genetic makeup, then logically, weight could be a matter of our DNA as well.

The nurture camp, by contrast, believes that obesity is a consequence of our surroundings and how we are raised— essentially, how our parents fed us, what they taught us to eat, how much they encouraged us to exercise, and the environment we lived in. Maybe, mom let us have too much soda and sugary cereal when we were kids, and now we don't know how to eat healthfully as adults. Or maybe, mom and dad worked too much and let TV serve as a babysitter, leaving little opportunity for playtime outside. Maybe, grandpa and grandma owned a candy or ice cream store when we were growing up. After all, who better to blame anything on than our family?

So which camp is correct? Should we blame mom and dad for giving us bad genes? Or for teaching us bad behaviors? Is it nature or nurture? Neither? Both? Before we answer this question, let us agree that this debate completely oversimplifies the issue. Obesity has *hundreds* of different possible causes, and although we may prefer to boil down these causes into a few important pathways (e.g., genetic vs. environmental), it is essentially an impossible feat.

The Nature Camp

For anyone who has opened the book randomly to this spot, this section is not about a summer camp specializing in nature hikes and microscopes; rather, it provides a summary of the genetic causes of obesity. Sorry. The study of the genetic basis of obesity dates back more than 20 years. Back in 1986, Stunkard, Foch, and Hrubec reported that body mass indices (BMIs) were more similar for identical (monozygotic) twins than for fraternal (dizygotic) twins. Given that identical twins share 100% of their DNA, whereas fraternal twins share only about 50%, assuming they were raised in the same household, one could draw the conclusion that this added level of similarity in BMI for identical twins is an artifact of genetics and DNA. After all, if genes did not determine obesity, then the identical twins should be no more similar than the fraternal twins. More recent studies have reported that the concordance of obesity for identical twins is 74% as compared with 32% for fraternal twins (Cummings & Schwartz, 2003). (Concordance just refers to the degree of similarity. Now you can enjoy wowing your friends when you use it in a sentence.)

Twin Studies

Before we go further, it's important to recognize how twins provide an extremely unique and valuable asset to anyone researching genetics, in part because between twin studies and adoption studies, you can often tease out (to some degree at least) the impacts of environment and genetics. Identical twins share 100% of their DNA, and if they grow up together, they also share their environment. They were in the womb together, they were raised together at the same time, they go to the same schools, probably had many of the same teachers, share the same clothes, watch the same shows, probably eat many of the same foods and meals together, maybe even dated the same people, etc. Fraternal twins share 50% of DNA, and also share a very similar environment if they grow up together. Siblings several years apart share 50% of their DNA, but usually have slightly less similar environments than fraternal twins. Children growing up in households with adopted siblings do not share DNA, but they *do* share an environment. And finally, we can look at twins or siblings who have been separated at birth as they share DNA but grew up in different environments. When comparing these groups ranging across the spectrum in genetic similarity and environmental similarity, we can begin to make some sense of the nature vs. nurture landscape.

Some may think that the high concordance rate among identical twins reported above (74%) is inflated because they share so much of their environment and life experiences. So to dig a little deeper, we look at close relatives who were raised in different environments due to adoption or separation from the family. Some early research found that adopted children more closely resembled their biological parents in weight than their adoptive parents (Stunkard et al., 1986). Stunkard, Harris, Pedersen, and McClearn (1990) later studied an even better sample of identical and fraternal twins who had been reared apart or together. The correlations in BMI for identical twins reared apart were .70 for men and .66 for women,[1] which is remarkably similar to those found among identical twins reared in the same household. These findings would suggest that their DNA had a stronger impact than the environment because the concordance rate remained high even when the environment was modified.

BOX 2.1 A PRIMER IN GENETIC TERMINOLOGY

Monozygotic = identical twins, share 100% of their DNA.

Dizygotic = fraternal twins, share approximately 50% of their DNA.

Monogenetic = caused by a mutation in a single gene.

Polygenetic = caused by many different gene variants in combination often acting in tandem with each other and the environment.

Genomics = the study of the entire human genome, including single genes and interactions between genes and the environment.

Epigenetics = the study of heritable changes in the genome that are not a function of a change in DNA sequence. These can involve changes to DNA structure and gene expression, including things such as DNA methylation, histone methylation chromatin modification, and genomic imprinting (Campion et al., 2009; Gluckman & Hanson, 2008; Walley et al., 2009).

Heritability

One way of quantifying the degree that genes contribute to BMI is through heritability estimates. Heritability, in this context, refers to the proportion of variance in BMI that can be attributed to genetic variance among individuals in a certain population. (Heritability is often reported as ranging from 0 to 1, but for ease of interpretation it is also expressed as a percent.)

Still confused? That's alright; heritability is a very confusing concept, so let us spend some time describing what exactly a "heritability estimate of 70%" means.[2] We can start with defining variance. Without getting into too much statistical mumbo-jumbo, variance helps us quantify how much variation exists for a given characteristic among a given population. If we are looking at the variance of height among U.S. women, for example, we know that the average height is 5′4″, but if you were to take a sample of 100 women, you would have considerable variation around that average. Some women might be 5′8″; others might be 5′2″. To calculate the variance in height among this sample of 100 women, you would take each woman's height and calculate the difference between the average height (5′4″), and then square that difference. Add up all of those values for each woman in the sample and you have the total variance in observed height.

Back to heritability, if we calculate the variance in BMI (obesity) in a given sample of individuals, then we know that a certain percentage of this variance will be due to variation in genes between individuals in our sample, a certain percentage will be due to variation in other environmental factors, and some will be due to covariance (which, in short, takes into account the relationship between genes and environment). You can see how the variance is divided up in the following equation:

$$\text{Variance (Obesity)} = \text{Variance (Environment)}$$
$$+ \text{Variance (Genetics)} + \text{Covariance}$$
$$\text{(Genetics and Environment)}$$

We often calculate these percentages by looking at how similar identical twins are as compared with fraternal twins, or identical twins reared together compared with identical twins reared apart, and so forth. This helps us estimate how much of the variance in BMI is due to the overall variation in genetic makeup in our sample and how much is due to variation in environments.

Across a range of twin studies, the heritability of obesity has fallen somewhere between 30% and 85% (Bulik, Sullivan, & Kendler, 2003; Herbert et al., 2006; Loos & Bouchard, 2003; Malis et al., 2005; Romeis, Grant, Knopik, Pedersen, & Heath, 2004; Schousboe et al., 2003; Wardle, Carnell, Haworth, & Plomin, 2008). Heritability estimates of other factors related to obesity are also fairly high:

- Dietary intake (i.e., eating habits); about 42% (De Castro, 2004)
- Percent body fat; 63% to 64% (Elder et al., 2008)
- Rate of change in BMI over time; approximately 58% to 64% (Hjelmborg et al., 2008)
- Appetite-related traits such as satiety responsiveness (i.e., how attuned you are to feeling full) and enjoyment of food; 63% and 75%, respectively (Wardle & Carnell, 2009)
- Physical activity; 55% (Mustelin, Silventoinen, Pietilainen, Rissanen, & Kaprio, 2008)

Problems with Heritability Estimates

Before you get too excited at the prospect of officially closing the nature vs. nurture debate, let us draw your attention to some of the misconceptions or critiques of using heritability estimates (in no particular order).

1. A heritability of 70% does NOT mean that the trait is 70% due to genetics and 30% due to the environment. Instead, heritability refers to how *genetic variation* relates to *observed variation* in a particular outcome (in this case obesity), but does *not* mean that genes are responsible for a specified degree of that outcome. This is probably the most common misinterpretation of heritability, and may be a large contributing factor to the disagreement and misunderstandings within the nature vs. nurture argument. In other words, you cannot go call your mom and tell her that her weight is 70% due to her genes (or worse yet, call her and blame her for passing on her genes to you). Nor can you say that 70% of obesity in the United States is because of our genes. The correct (and only) interpretation of the heritability estimates across a range of studies is that between 30% and 85% of the variation in BMI can be attributed to genetic variance.

   Say, for example, that we wanted to look at the impact of dog breed on aggression. If we were to find heritability estimates of 75% for aggression in dogs, we would interpret this to mean that 75% of the variation in aggression (i.e., how much variance there is in our sample for number of dog fights) can be attributed to the genetic variance across different dog breeds. It would not tell us what breeds are aggressive, which genes lead to dog fights, or the particular balance of genes and poor training that leads a dog to become aggressive. This brings us to our second point.

2. Heritability does NOT tell you anything about the average BMI, just how individuals vary around that average. Recall that variance is simply the sum of squared deviations from the mean. So the fact that the variance in BMI may be explained largely by genetic variation says nothing about why the mean BMI has increased over time, or why the mean BMI may be different between populations. Heritability also tells us nothing about specific genes (or specific environmental factors) that contribute to individual variation in BMI.

3. Heritability estimates are NOT universal, and are specific only to a particular group at a particular time within particular environments. One would likely not find the same level of heritability across all populations and environments. In fact, heritability estimates can change over time even within the same group of people. Heritability of BMI has been found to increase from 56% at age 4, to 64% at age 7, to 78% at age 10 (Haworth, Plomin, Carnell, & Wardle, 2008). The take-home message is that the studies using twin registries in Denmark produce heritability estimates that are relevant only to that population of twins living in Denmark at that time. It is not applicable to a population of Ugandan children born in 2000, or to a population of American adults living in Kansas in 1905. These different populations would have different variances in BMI, genetic makeup, and environments, and would therefore have different heritability estimates. This is one possible explanation for why heritability estimates have ranged so much in the literature, from 30% to more than 85%.

4. A related issue is that if you have very little environmental variation, because your entire sample consists of twins living in Liverpool, England, in 1994, for example, you will end up with artificially high heritability estimates. When using the equation above, low environment variance will likely lead to a high heritability estimate. Conversely, if there is little genetic variation, then heritability will be artificially low. Take for example, the fact that humans are born with two eyes. We know this trait is genetic. It is in almost everyone's DNA (save the very rare mutation and the sci-fi thriller "The Fly"). However, if you calculate the heritability of having two eyes using the equation above, it will be exceptionally low (maybe close to zero). This is because almost all of the variation in having two eyes among people is environmental (e.g., people have accidents with nail-guns or bows and arrows). So you end up with a heritability estimate that is extremely low, despite the fact that having two eyes is clearly determined by genes. This is because variance and heritability estimates only help in explaining *variation* within the population rather than helping appoint blame.

   Within the context of obesity, some people have said that we have simply reached a point where our environment is so "obesogenic," meaning an environment that is universally conducive to weight gain, that there really is no significant variation (Ravussin & Bogardus, 2000; Silventoinen, Rokholm, Kaprio, & Sorensen, 2010). When candy and fast food is never more than two minutes away, how much variation is there? This may contribute to a relatively high heritability estimates, despite large environmental contributions to obesity.

5. Finally, Schonemann (1997) reported problems with estimating heritability using twin studies, as he found that responses to the question "Did you have your back rubbed last year?" were 92% heritable for males, and 21% for females. It is unclear how receiving a back rub in the past year would

be highly heritable for males, so suffice it to say, heritability estimates should be viewed with caution.

The Nurture Camp

With a bit of simple math, you might realize that if 30% to 85% of the variability in BMI is due to genetic variation, and covariance is assumed to be 0 (it usually is assumed to be 0, which can also be problematic), then somewhere between 15% and 70% is due to variation in environments. Other research has reported that 58% of the variance in dietary intake, 72% of the variation in meal size, and 64% of the variation in meal frequency is due to variation in the environment (De Castro, 2004). There are many other pieces of compelling evidence for the environmental causes of obesity. We will discuss many of these later in this chapter.

Some striking evidence that the environment plays a large role in obesity stemmed from research on the Pima Indians. The Pima Indians living in Arizona have some of the highest rates of obesity and non-insulin-dependent diabetes mellitus in the world (Ravussin, Valencia, Esparza, Bennett, & Schulz, 1994). There is a population related to the Pima Indians of Arizona, living in northwestern Mexico, that instead maintains an average BMI in the normal range. These two groups share a gene pool, but have very different lifestyles (Schulz et al., 2006). The Pimas living in Arizona follow a "westernized" lifestyle of high-fat diets and low levels of physical activity. The Mexican Pimas, by contrast, live in a remote mountainous region with a lifestyle closer to our ancestors—they grow and farm their own food, perform high levels of manual labor, live largely without technology (no wireless, 3D plasma TVs, or even cars). The mean BMI of Mexican Pimas was 24.9 kg/m^2 (±4.0 kg/m^2) compared with 33.4 kg/m^2 (±7.5 kg/m^2) for the Arizona Pimas (Ravussin et al., 1994). A more recent study of the same populations reported even greater differences in obesity. Less than 7% of Mexican Pima men, and 19.8% of Mexican Pima women were obese, compared with 63.8% of Arizona Pima men and 74.8% of Arizona Pima women (Schulz et al., 2006). That means that the Arizona Pima men were almost 10 times more likely to be obese than the Mexican Pima men! Because these groups share a gene pool, this huge increase in risk of obesity appears to be largely due to differences in their lifestyles and environments.

Other studies have shown that risk of obesity increases for immigrants moving from other countries to the United States, and that risk of obesity increases through the generations. In other words, second-generation immigrants are more likely to be obese than their parents, third-generation immigrants are more likely to be obese than their parents, and so on (Bates, Acevedo-Garcia, Alegria, & Krieger, 2006; Popkin & Udry, 1998). Among immigrant subgroups, those who have spent more time living in the United States are more likely to be obese than those who immigrated to the United States more recently (Barcenas et al., 2007; Sanghavi-Goel, McCarthy, Phillips, & Wee, 2004). Only 8% of those living in the United States for less than 1 year were obese, compared with 19% of those living in the United States for more than 15 years (Sanghavi-Goel et al., 2004). Another study of Hispanic immigrants reported similar findings; only 9% of those living in the United States for less than 4 years were obese, compared with 24.2% of those living in the United States for more than 15 years (Kaplan, Huguet, Newsom, & McFarland, 2004). Perhaps, the new U.S. slogan should be "the land of opportunity... to become obese."

If the human genome has not changed much in the past 10,000 years, then it surely has not changed much over three generations of immigrants to the United States. Therefore, it must be environmental factors that are driving these large increases in obesity among U.S. immigrant populations. Large environmental influences on obesity are further supported by studies demonstrating a wide range of obesity prevalence estimates among 34 different countries around the world. Children from Malta and the United States were most likely to be obese, whereas children from Lithuania and Latvia were least likely to be obese (Janssen et al., 2005). Other comparisons have shown that obesity is much more common in economically developed countries (Kelly, Yang, Chen, Reynolds, & He, 2008; Prentice, 2006). The prevalence of obesity in the United States has been the highest in the world, though the prevalence of obesity is rising in both developed and developing nations around the globe (Hossain, Kawar, & El Nahas, 2007; Kelly et al., 2008; World Health Organization, 2000) as they adopt "Western" life-styles of decreased physical activity and higher consumption of cheap, calorie-dense foods (Hossain et al., 2007). Calorie-dense refers to foods that have a large number of calories in a relatively small volume of food. For example, a cup of cookie dough packs a lot more calories than a cup of watermelon or a cup of celery sticks. For a discussion of what "healthy food" means, see Box 2.2.

BOX 2.2 WHAT IS "HEALTHY FOOD" ANYWAY?

Throughout this book, we often refer to "healthy" or "unhealthy" food. You might have noticed the last time you were in a grocery store that there was no dividing line down the middle with "healthy food" on one side and "unhealthy food" on the other. You probably didn't see brightly colored labels on all of the items marking some as healthy and some as unhealthy. (Though some food producers have created their own labels, such as check marks or other symbols of supposed healthfulness, you certainly didn't see a skull and crossbones on any candy bars.) Even in the aisles that seem to contain mostly "healthy foods," you might find a box of granola that is deceptively high in fat and calories. Lumping products together into "healthy food" or "unhealthy food" catego-ries is a bit like trying to sort the American population

BOX 2.2 CONTINUED

into groups of "tall people" and "short people." At the extremes, it is easy to determine who fits in which category. Certainly, a person who is 6'6" is tall, and a person who is 5'0" is short. However, what about all the people in between? Similarly, we can be pretty confident in saying that carrots and spinach are healthy and super-chocolate-peanut-butter-caramel ice cream is unhealthy. But most food products fall somewhere in between. Additionally, context matters. If the average height in the population is 6'4", then maybe 6'6" isn't really that tall. If someone eats mostly nutritious, fresh fruits and vegetables, lean meats, and whole grains, then most nutritionists would say the occasional hot-fudge sundae is fine. Conversely, if someone eats primarily fried food, then the occasional bite of broccoli is not going to be sufficient (especially if the broccoli is also fried). So when we refer to "healthy food" or "healthy diet," what we are really talking about is an overall dietary pattern that is consistent with what nutritionists have been recommending for decades: an appropriate number of calories coming from plenty of fresh fruits and vegetables, whole grains, lean proteins, with little saturated fat and added sugar. An unhealthy diet, by contrast, is typically full of energy-dense foods (read: high in fat and added sugars) that pack a lot of calories but very little nutritional value. These terms are not meant to demonize or lionize any particular food or type of food. Even fast-food outlets have healthy options nowadays, and vegetarians can have unhealthy diets too.

Even looking at differences within the United States, we find that there is tremendous variation across the states with respect to prevalence of obesity (Bethell, Simpson, Stumbo, Carle, & Gombojav, 2010; Chou, Grossman, & Saffer, 2004). It is hard to see how there would be significant genetic differences between the people living in Colorado, as compared with Mississippi, so these differences in obesity prevalence are assumed to be largely due to variations in environments and lifestyles.

It's completely understandable for you to be scratching your head wondering "So which is it then? Genes or environment?" There seems to be a compelling case for each side of the argument; hence, the ongoing nature vs. nature debate. However, as you will see in the next section, the nature/nurture divide is really a false dichotomy. It tragically oversimplifies an exceedingly complex issue, and to be quite honest, it does not make a whole lot of sense. If you keep reading (you've made it this far!), you'll see why.

Our Evolution Toward Obesity

To truly understand why so many people are obese now, we have to look back 10,000 years to our ancestors. Although the average first-grader may not realize it, humans did not always live in a world where food could be found 100 feet away in the nearest vending machine. Our ancestors had to survive in an environment in which food was scarce, and famine was a part of life. They also had to expend tremendous energy to hunt and gather food. In other words, our ancestors alternated between periods of rest and intense physical activity, as well as feast and famine (Chakravarthy & Booth, 2004). Overindulgence, two-for-one sales at the bakery, and holiday potlucks were luxuries they could not afford or comprehend. It is thought that humans adapted to this lifestyle by becoming more and more efficient at storing energy (i.e., excess calories were stored as fat; Bellisari, 2008; Chakravarthy & Booth, 2004; Gardner & Rhodes, 2009). They built up fat reserves when food was plentiful, equipping them with energy to utilize while searching for food, helping them weather the cold season, and giving them a reserve of energy to deplete during famines. During this period in our ancient history, it is thought that certain "thrifty genotypes" evolved, where individuals who were particularly adept at obtaining (through physical activity) and storing food (as fat) were more likely to survive and procreate (Neel, 1962). Now, one point of clarification, the term "thrifty genotype" refers to several genes that influence a host of bodily functions related to metabolism, diet, activity, and weight (among other things), not a singular gene.

This is a prime example of the processes of evolution and natural selection at work. Thrifty genes evolved, and these genes turned some humans into well-oiled energy storing machines. These humans then had a great survival advantage during periods of famine or food scarcity and were able to pass on the thrifty genotype to subsequent generations. It should be said that there is not 100% consensus that this is how history unfolded. There is another theory that "genetic drift" and "predation release" caused obesity to simply become neutral to our ancestors, as opposed to detrimental (Speakman, 2004). Here, the theory goes that it was disadvantageous to be too thin (because you might starve to death) and it was disadvantageous to be obese (because you have more trouble evading predators) for a long period of human history. At some point, millions of years ago, humans evolved past the threat of predation—we developed social behavior, mastered fire, made weapons, and so on. At that point, it no longer became disadvantageous to be overweight or obese. Our genome subsequently "drifted" toward higher body weights.

Although we can't know for sure how the genetic lottery played out in early human history, one thing is largely agreed upon today: our current population is cursed with the highly efficient, energy storing genetic legacy of our ancient relatives. You might be surprised to learn that in the past 10,000 years, there have been astoundingly few changes to the human genome (Chakravarthy & Booth, 2004). What have changed over the past 10,000 years, however, are our lifestyles and environments.

So maybe you can't blame mom and dad for your weight, but you can blame mom and dad's great grandparents,

6,000 times removed, right? Not quite. As you might have guessed by now, the picture is a bit more complicated.

Genes and Environment: A Nonexclusive Relationship

Gene–environment interactions are when the effects of a gene (or combination of genes) are greater in the presence of certain environmental factors, and vice versa. For example, a person may have a certain risk for cardiovascular disease (CVD) based on his or her genes. This risk is compounded by exposure to smoke (either through that person smoking, or exposure to second-hand smoke). This person's genes *interact* with his or her environment to greatly increase the risk of CVD. Alcoholism is another example, as there is both a genetic component and an environmental component, and outcomes can differ depending on whether you join a fraternity or join a seminary. Gene–environment interactions are being researched, and many have been identified. Certain genes are expressed (or not) depending upon various environmental exposures or lifestyle factors, such as physical activity or high-fat diets (Clement, 2005).

As an example, say we are interested in the genetic and environmental causes of freckles. Intuitively, we know that some people develop freckles, and others do not. We also know that sun exposure leads to freckles, and the more you are in the sun, the more freckles you will have. If we look at a population of lifeguards at a Tahitian beach (i.e., they all have similarly high levels of sun exposure), then we would find that genetics must determine who gets freckles and who does not. If everyone has the same sun exposure, then obviously genetics is what differentiates the freckled from the smoothly tanned. However, if we are looking at a population of people who are entirely nocturnal (i.e., vampires), then no one will develop freckles (or tans, for that matter). The paleness of these individuals is completely determined by their environment. You can see in this example that a person's genes interact with his or her environment to cause freckles. For any given individuals, the number of freckles they have is a combination of their genetic predisposition and their environmental exposures.

Now imagine that we told you that the average number of freckles on any given person had increased by 20% over the past 50 years. Or that the percentage of people with freckles has increased by 300% over the same time period. You would likely conclude that there is something about our environment that is causing this societal shift, because our genetic predisposition for freckles could not possibly have changed that quickly.

This example really gets to the crux of the nature vs. nurture debate. The nature camp and the nurture camp are really focused on two different questions. The nature camp is seeking to answer the question, "What makes some people obese, and others underweight if we are all exposed to this obesogenic environment?" To answer this question, we look to heritability estimates to tell us about individual variation in BMI. The nurture camp, by contrast, is really seeking to answer the questions, "Why are so many people now obese compared with 50 years ago? Why is obesity more prevalent among some groups than others that presumably have very similar genetic make-ups?" To answer these questions, heritability estimates are completely useless. We need to look at how our society has changed over time, or how lifestyles and environments differ between groups. As two leading researchers put it:

> Among different populations, the prevalence of obesity is largely determined by environmental factors. However, among individuals from the same population, living in a given environment, the variability in body size and body composition is mostly related to genetically determined response to that environment. (Ravussin & Bogardus, 2000, p. S17)

Hopefully now you can see that the nature vs. nurture debate is a fairly useless and misguided one, at least when viewing them independent or mutually exclusive of one another.

Both genetics and environment play very large, often overlapping roles, in causing obesity.

SO WHAT CAUSES OBESITY?

Fundamentally, obesity is a consequence of caloric imbalance. Caloric balance is achieved when energy intake equals energy expenditure. In other words, when we take in the same number of calories as we use up, we have caloric balance. Caloric *imbalance* occurs when we take in a greater number of calories than we use up, resulting in weight gain and eventually obesity; or when we take in fewer calories than we burn, resulting in weight loss and eventually underweight. When we consume excess calories, they get stored as fat (regardless of whether the calories originally came from protein, fat, or carbohydrates; if there are extra calories, they get stored in the body as fat). Our bodies do try to compensate and adjust for over- or under-consumption by changing how many calories we burn. If we starve ourselves, then our metabolisms slow down to compensate,[3] much like our ancestors whose bodies became efficient at storing energy. Conversely, if we overeat by a few calories, then our bodies expend a bit more energy to make up for this imbalance. At some point, our bodies can no longer compensate for the extra energy we are taking in, so that extra then gets stored as fat. An extra 3,500 calories is equivalent to one pound. Roughly, an extra 500 calories each day will result in a one-pound weight gain over a week. On the other hand, if you were to take up long-distance running and burn an extra 500 calories per day, you would lose one pound per week. (These numbers are a little fuzzy because they do not take into account the fact that your body compensates for part of the imbalance, but you get the idea).

To maintain our weights, we have to walk the tightrope balancing energy intake on one side and energy expenditure on the other. This balancing act is called energy homeostasis. Total energy expenditure is made up of several components. Resting metabolic rate is the largest component, representing 80% of all energy expenditure (Landsberg, Young, Leonard, Linsenmeier, & Turek, 2009). This is essentially what your body would burn if you slept all day long. The thermic effect of food is the energy burned to digest food (about 10%). Physical activity is a relatively small component of overall energy expenditure, accounting for about another 10% (Landsberg et al., 2009). Obviously, if you are running ultramarathons, this percentage will increase. You can see that you basically have two options for adjusting the balancing act: (1) change how many calories you take in or (2) change how many calories you burn through physical activity.

It turns out that for most of human history, we were pretty good at walking this tightrope. Most normal-weight people gain about 0.5 to 1 lb per year during their adult lives (Fox, 1973; Schmitz, Jacobs, Leon, Schreiner, & Sternfeld, 2000; Sternfeld et al., 2004). Most overweight people gain about 2 to 3 lbs per year over their adult lives (McPherson, 2007; Schmitz et al., 2000). Unfortunately, even very small imbalances can result in large weight gains over long periods of time.

Researchers have looked at how big the "energy gap" between caloric intake and energy expenditure would have to be to explain the rising prevalence in obesity in the United States. The estimates vary, but it seems that an excess intake of between 20 and 245 calories per day would explain why the prevalence of obesity has risen so drastically in the United States over the past several decades (Brown, Williams, Ford, Ball, & Dobson, 2005; Butte & Ellis, 2003; Hill, Wyatt, Reed, & Peters, 2003; Plachta-Danielzik et al., 2008; Wang, Gortmaker, Sobol, & Kuntz, 2006). By one report, if adults in the United States cut their caloric intake by about 100 calories each day, this would be sufficient to stop weight gain for approximately 90% of the U.S. population (Hill et al., 2003). For normal-weight children, they would have to cut out 100 to 165 calories each day to stop excessive weight gain (Butte & Ellis, 2003; Plachta-Danielzik et al., 2008; Wang et al., 2006). To halt weight gain for 90% of overweight children, they would need to cut out somewhere between 200 and 1,017 calories each day (Butte & Ellis, 2003; Wang et al., 2006). In other words, if most of the population could cut out a can of sugar-sweetened soda, or two cookies, or two slices of cheese, or a handful of small pretzels, or even just ¼ of a bagel (all approximately 100 calories) each day, we could make a huge dent in the obesity epidemic in the United States. For those at higher risk for weight gain over time, such as overweight children, the cuts would have to be larger to prevent weight gain over time.

The Cellular Level

Humans are born with a certain number of fat cells (adipocytes), and this number grows fairly rapidly after birth and during puberty. Aside from those growth periods, the number of fat cells in the body is fairly static, at least among weight-stable people (Fruhbeck, 2008; Spalding et al., 2008; van Harmelen et al., 2003). Energy imbalance and the accumulation of fat results in the fat cells getting larger rather than increasing in number (Drolet et al., 2008; Fruhbeck, 2008; Walley, Asher, & Froguel, 2009). However, at a certain critical point, the cells can no longer expand, and are forced to divide and form new fat cells (Faust, Johnson, Stern, & Hirsh, 1978; Jo et al., 2009; van Harmelen et al., 2003). I'm sure many of us wish our stomachs could do this after Thanksgiving dinner.

As you might expect, obese individuals have both a greater number of fat cells as well as larger-sized fat cells than normal-weight individuals (Cinti, 2005; Coppack, 2005; Drolet et al., 2008; Spalding et al., 2008). Moreover, obese individuals have a greater number of fat cells added each year (8,000,000,000 new cells per year) compared with normal-weight individuals (3,000,000,000 new fat cells per year, probably a consequence of normal cell turnover; Spalding et al., 2008). One study using rats proposed that increases in fat cell size are due primarily to diet, whereas increases in fat cell number are a combination of diet and genetics (Jo et al., 2009). Some research on obese individuals who had early (childhood) onset of obesity has found that increases in fat cell number occur only during growth periods in youth (Drolet et al., 2008; Spalding et al., 2008), and that during adulthood, fat cells increase in size but not in number. This suggests that there are sensitive windows of development where children are at particular risk for the irreversible accumulation of body fat. We refer to this as irreversible because once you reach a certain number of fat cells, you can't get rid of them, even if you lose weight (except through liposuction or some other surgery where fat is removed). Fat cells can decrease in size from exercise and diet, but not in number (Spalding et al., 2008). This makes it particularly difficult to get back to your ideal weight once you have gained a substantial amount, especially for those who experienced a significant growth in fat cells during childhood. Depressing, right?

To sum up, our ancestors passed on thrifty genes, which turned out to be pretty maladaptive in our current obesogenic environment, putting us at increased risk for obesity. Whereas individual differences in weight status may be largely due to genes, our environment is responsible for group differences and the overall rise in prevalence of obesity over time.

Now, on to the specifics.

GENETIC CAUSES OF OBESITY

Few research topics capture the public's imagination like the search for genes that predispose to obesity...However, it is clear that complex diseases such as obesity are not caused by genes alone, but involve interplay between genetics, diet, infectious agents, environment, behavior, and social structures. (Pomp & Mohlke, 2008, p. 36)

Astronomical sums of money and amounts of time have been spent researching the genetic causes of obesity. Mapping the human genome has propelled the field forward in recent years. Currently, there have been more than 600 genes or markers associated with obesity (Rankinen et al., 2006; Snyder et al., 2004). There are also several genetic syndromes that are associated with obesity, including Prader-Willi, Cohen, Alstrom, Carpenter's, and Bardet-Biedl syndromes. Still, other medical conditions, such as underactive thyroid, can result in weight gain and obesity; however, these conditions are rare. If you are interested in more details about specific genes, see The Human Obesity Gene Map (Rankinen et al., 2006).

The genetic causes of obesity are often separated into to two types: monogenic and polygenic. Monogenic obesity refers to forms of obesity that result from very rare mutations in single genes. These forms are typically evident very early in life and are very severe. The second form, polygenic obesity, refers to several genetic variants that interact with each other (and with the environment). In the case of polygenic obesity, any single gene susceptibility would have a very small effect, but taken together, the cumulative effect of several susceptibilities (perhaps in combination with environmental factors) leads to a substantially increased risk of obesity.

Monogenic Causes of Obesity

The single gene mutations responsible for obesity (at least those identified so far) are mostly associated with appetite (O'Rahilly, Farooqi, Yeo, & Challis, 2003). More specifically, these gene mutations typically affect the *leptin* and *melanocortin* pathways, which are critical for weight homeostasis, controlling satiety (feelings of fullness) and food intake (hunger; O'Rahilly & Farooqi, 2006).

There are several other genes and mutations that have been identified, but these are exceedingly rare. To give you a sense of how rare, a "common" variant of the FTO gene (a gene that has been linked to obesity) accounts for less than 1% of the heritability of BMI (Frayling et al., 2007; Walley et al., 2009). Another mutation called MC4R has been thought to account for only 0.5% to 2% of moderate obesity cases and only 4% of severe obesity (Crowley, 2008; Santini et al., 2009). Despite such low numbers, these mutations are the most common genetic causes of obesity.

All in all, it is estimated that single gene mutations account for only 1% to 5% of cases of obesity (Loos & Bouchard, 2003; Newell, Zlot, Silvey, & Ariail, 2007). That means out of 100 obese people, somewhere between 1 and 5 will have some kind of genetic mutation that causes them to be obese. That said, even among those with genetic abnormalities that cause obesity, the effect of environment is not negligible as there is still variation in body weight that suggests other factors also contribute to obesity.

Polygenic Causes of Obesity

There are many genes that interact with each other and with the environment to influence the energy equation. For example, we have genes that influence hunger or appetite, eating frequency, satiety or fullness, taste for different foods, physical activity, metabolism, inflammation, thermogenesis, fat tissue development, and so on (Booth & Shanely, 2004; Chakravarthy & Booth, 2004; Christodoulides et al., 2006; Coughlin et al., 2007; Farooqi & O'Rahilly, 2007; Herbert et al., 2006; Loos et al., 2005, 2007; Moran et al., 2006; Mutch & Clement, 2006; Simonen et al., 2003; Stone et al., 2006; Tankó et al., 2005; van Erk et al., 2006). Energy balance or homeostasis is influenced by many different physiological factors, including hormones and peptides (e.g., ghrelin, peptide YY, leptin, adinoponectin, cholecystokinin, neuropeptide Y, melanin-concentrating hormone, agouti-related peptide, corticotropin-releasing hormone, insulin), neurotransmitters such as serotonin, and various body organs, such as the gut, pancreas, and hypothalamus

(Cummings & Schwartz, 2003; Levin, 2009; Paracchini, Pedotti, & Taioli, 2005; Walley et al., 2009). Any one disruption to these functions may have a relatively small effect; but many genetic factors can all add together to greatly increase the chances that a person will be obese. Environmental factors add to these genetic risk factors as well. It is now pretty much agreed upon (at least in academic circles) that, "in most cases, obesity is characterized by the strong interaction of genetic and environmental factors over time with a strong polygenic contribution (Romao & Roth, 2008)" (Bluher, 2009, p. 242). Any one of these factors alone may only be responsible for a few hundred grams of body weight, making them exceptionally hard to detect (Hebebrand & Hinney, 2009).

Prenatal and Early Childhood Exposures

Parent Weight and Obesity

Children of two obese parents are more than 10 times more likely to be obese than children with normal-weight parents (Reilly et al., 2005). It's hard to say, however, whether children have inherited a genetic propensity for obesity (as discussed above) or a set of habits (as will be discussed below), although it's likely a little of both.

Prenatal Exposures and Obesity

Similar to the "thrifty genotype" hypothesis described above, a "thrifty phenotype" hypothesis has been proposed to explain findings that certain exposures in utero are associated with obesity (Hales & Barker, 1992). The baby adapts to his or her environment in the womb, and these metabolic adaptations can become permanent (on the up side, they can be reversed as well). Even very early life experiences (in the womb or immediately postbirth) can make long-lasting changes to our hard-wired DNA (Prentice, 2005) that influence how genes are expressed, and these changes can be passed on to subsequent generations (Campion, Milagro, & Martinez, 2009; Newnham, Pennell, Lye, Rampono, & Challis, 2009).

For example, insufficient fetal nutrition has been associated with lower birth weights and subsequent obesity (Gluckman & Hanson, 2008; Levin, 2009). In other words, if the mother eats too little and does not gain sufficient weight during her pregnancy, her offspring are at higher risk for obesity in the future. This has been hypothesized to be a result of compensatory or "catch-up" growth after nutritional restriction, or the consequence of epigenetic processes (Gluckman & Hanson, 2008; Newnham et al., 2009).

On the flip side, excessive maternal weight gain during pregnancy is also associated with obesity (Newnham et al., 2009). Regardless of pre-pregnancy body mass, excessive weight gain during pregnancy is positively associated with the risk of obesity among children at age 3 years (Oken, Taveras, Kleinman, Rich-Edwards, & Gillman, 2007). Some of this relationship may be due to the fact that large birth weights are associated with obesity for that child later on (Martorell, Stein, & Schroeder, 2001; Newnham et al., 2009), and mothers who gain more weight during pregnancy tend to have larger babies (duh). Additionally, maternal obesity during pregnancy (regardless of weight gain) demonstrates a strong relationship with obesity during childhood. Nearly one in four preschool children (24%) of mothers who were obese in the first trimester was obese, as compared with 9% of children born to mothers who were normal weight (Whitaker, 2004). Combined with research suggesting that inadequate nutrition in utero also may lead to obesity, it seems that mothers who gain too little or too much weight during pregnancy are at increased risk for having obese children. As if there wasn't enough pressure on pregnant women to begin with.

Other health conditions, such as gestational diabetes (when a woman develops diabetes during pregnancy), have been associated with obesity among children and adolescents, as high fetal insulin levels can promote fat cell development in utero and rapid weight gain after birth (Gillman, Rifas-Shiman, Berkey, Field, & Colditz, 2003; Gluckman & Hanson, 2008).

Maternal stress during pregnancy has also been associated with small newborn size and may have implications for child weight status (Newnham et al., 2009). Maternal smoking during pregnancy has also been associated with childhood obesity (Oken, Levitan, & Gillman, 2008).

Not only can gene expression be altered by in-utero experiences to increase the risk of obesity but also neural pathways can be affected as well (Levin, 2009). The parts of the baby's brain that control appetite (i.e., certain functions of the hypothalamus) are relatively plastic in early life and are affected by factors such as maternal nutrition (i.e., mom eating too much during pregnancy) or overfeeding of the infant after birth (Gluckman & Hanson, 2008).

Habits of Early Childhood and Obesity

Rapid weight gain during infancy is associated with obesity in adulthood (Baird et al., 2005; Monteiro & Victoria, 2005; Ong & Loos, 2006; Reilly et al., 2005; Stettler, 2007). Babies who are formula fed tend to grow faster than those who are breast fed (Gluckman & Hanson, 2008). This may contribute to the finding that breast feeding is protective against obesity (Harder, Bergmann, Kallischnigg, & Plagemann, 2005; Owen et al., 2005). Going too far toward the other extreme can pose a risk too; restricting the food intake of infants is associated with risk of obesity at age 3 (Taveras et al., 2006).

Sleeping too little in the first years of life is also related to obesity (Bell, Zimmerman, 2010; Reilly et al., 2005). One study found that fewer hours of sleep between the ages of 6 months and 2 years was associated with greater risk of obesity at 3 years (Taveras, Rifas-Shiman, Oken, Gunderson, & Gillman, 2008). Other factors in early life, such as TV watching, soda intake, and fast-food intake, as you might expect, are associated with later obesity (Reilly et al., 2005; Taveras, Gillman, Kleinman, Rich-Edwards, & Rifas-Shiman, 2010; Welsh et al., 2005). These factors are more common among some racial and ethnic subpopulations, setting these groups up for higher rates of obesity beginning in early childhood (Taveras et al., 2010).

Excess weight for kids younger than 2 years can put them at risk for subsequent obesity. Among a study of overweight or obese children (average age 12 years), half of them became overweight before 2 years of age, and 90% were overweight by 5 years of age (Harrington et al., 2010). Although many parents think that children will grow out of their "baby fat" (Etelson, Brand, Patrick, & Shirali, 2003; He & Evans, 2007), this is not usually the case (Nader et al., 2005). About 60% of kids who were overweight in preschool and 80% of kids who were overweight in elementary school went on to be overweight at age 12 (Nader et al., 2005). Even having a BMI in the top 50th percentile puts preschool children at risk for later obesity compared with children who have BMIs below the 50th percentile (Field, Cook, & Gillman, 2005). This is not to say that you should put your 2-year-old on a diet, but it does mean that healthy eating should start early to prevent excessive weight gain.

Not only does obesity in early childhood lead to obesity in adolescence but also obesity in adolescence leads to obesity in adulthood. Between 80% and 90% of overweight children between 10 and 15 years of age go on to become obese at 25 years of age (Guo, Wu, Chumlea, & Roche, 2002).

DIET AND ACTIVITY

As we discussed earlier in this chapter, weight gain and obesity are fundamentally a problem of energy imbalance. People take in more calories than they burn. Pretty much all of the identified causes of obesity operate by influencing either energy intake (diet) or energy expenditure (activity).

Diet

If you were to believe the claims made by the inventors of the latest diet crazes (FYI, you shouldn't), you might think that carbs (or fat, or protein, etc.) are evil one day and the cure for obesity the next. Despite the assertions of TV spokespeople trying to hawk their latest diet to you when you happen to be awake at 3:30 am, it is often said that, "a calorie is a calorie" (Bucholz & Schoeller, 2004). In other words, it does not matter whether the excess calories come from fat, protein, carbohydrates, or alcohol; if there are excess calories, they will end up in the body as fat. That being said, we know that there are significant nutritional differences between fat, protein, and carbohydrates.

It is easier to go overboard with dietary fat, because a gram of fat has nine calories, compared with four calories per gram for protein and carbohydrates (alcohol has seven calories per gram). Foods that are high in fat are typically what we call "energy dense" in that they pack a lot of calories in a small amount of food. Therefore, eating the same-sized portion of a food high in fat compared with a food high in protein will lead to more calories, and potentially higher probability of obesity for yourself and your progeny. There is some research in rats that has shown that a Western-like high-fat diet (i.e., 35% of calories from fat, with a certain makeup of fatty acids) can produce increases in body fat (both fat cell size and number) over several generations, even when total calories are constant (Massiera et al., 2010). If this relationship holds for humans as well, then it is possible that our Americanized high-fat diet could be contributing to obesity (and the steady increase across generations), but studies of this association are inconclusive (Melanson, Astrup, & Donahoo, 2009).

Most people believe that the high-fat diets contribute to obesity because they are exceptionally energy dense. Energy density is important because we feel full based on the volume or the weight of food that we eat, not how many calories are in it (Westerterp-Plantenga, 2004). In other words, two cups of salad will fill us up roughly the same as two cups of cookie dough, but the cookie dough packs a ton more calories than the salad. Our stomachs do not necessarily distinguish between foods that are energy dense or not. Our taste buds, however, do make this distinction. We tend to like the taste of energy dense foods (Kessler, 2009). Who wouldn't prefer a candy bar to a carrot stick? This may be a vestige of our thrifty genes. It would not have been very adaptive to our ancestors to prefer celery stalks to steaks when they are trying to survive long periods of food scarcity.

Although calories in any form will be stored as fat, there are differences in how full we feel after eating different types of nutrients. Namely, protein makes people feel fuller (so they may eat less), as does eating food with high water content or high fiber content (Buchholz & Schoeller, 2004; Schoeller & Buchholz, 2005; Westerterp-Plantenga, 2004). There is also some evidence that higher protein levels can boost metabolism (burning of calories) by a small amount (Buccholz & Schoeller, 2004). But at the end of the day, at least when it comes down to your weight, "a calorie is a calorie" still holds true (Buchholz & Schoeller, 2004). Excess calories, no matter where they come from, will result in excess fat.

So where do excess calories come from? There are so many answers to this question, we could literally write another whole book. Our eating patterns have changed dramatically over the past several decades, and many of these changes are thought to contribute to the rising prevalence of obesity in the United States. Here are a few ways in which our eating patterns have changed.

Restaurants, Fast Food, and Convenience

People are eating out more now than ever before. More than half of all food expenditures in the United States are spent outside the home, up from 34% in 1974 (Stewart, Blisard, & Jolliffe, 2006). Fast-food restaurants are the most popular option, accounting for half of all food consumed outside the home (St. Onge, Keller, & Heymsfield, 2003). Nearly one in three kids have fast food on any given day (Bowman, Gortmaker, Ebbeling, Pereira, & Ludwig, 2004), and 75% of teens have fast food at least once per week (French, Story, Neumark-Sztainer, Fulkerson, & Hannan, 2001).

The problem with eating out is that restaurant or fast food is higher in calories and total fat, and the portion sizes are larger than food served at home (Koplan et al., 2005). As such, Americans tend to consume nearly 200 more calories per day when they eat out compared with those who eat food prepared in the home (Frazao, 1999; Lin, Guthrie, & Frazao, 1999). Studies have shown that on the days that children eat fast food, they eat more calories, more fat, more sugar-sweetened drinks, and fewer fruits and vegetables (Bowman et al., 2004; Paeratakul, Ferdinand, Champagne, Ryan, & Bray, 2003). Other research has reported that on the days children consume fast food, they eat an excess of 187 calories (Brownell, 2004) and do not compensate for overconsumption of fast food by adjusting intake throughout the day or increasing activity level (Ebbeling et al., 2004). Over 1 year, this excess intake could produce a weight gain of six extra pounds, on average (Brownell, 2004). It should come as no surprise that regular fast-food consumption is a risk factor for obesity and weight gain (Agras & Mascola, 2005; Rosenheck, 2008).

Portion Sizes

One consequence of eating out so often is the exposure to huge portion sizes served at restaurants and fast-food places. Even ignoring "supersizing," portion sizes have increased dramatically in fast food and other restaurants (Ledikwe, Ello-Martin, & Rolls, 2005). There is some evidence that exposure to these enormous portions in restaurants leads us to prefer larger portions at home, too (Colapinto, Fitzgerald, Taper, & Veugelers, 2007). In effect, large portion sizes are normalized by eating out. At the same time portion sizes in restaurants have grown, portions at home have swelled, too, since the 1970s (Nielsen & Popkin, 2003).

Evidence that larger portion sizes have become normalized comes from a recent study looking at how big the supper was in paintings of The Last Supper. From some of the first paintings in 1,000 AD to present, the size of the entrée has increased by nearly 70% (Wansink & Wansink, 2010). Art really does imitate life.

It probably comes as no surprise that larger portion sizes are associated with higher caloric intake (Ledikwe et al., 2005) and obesity (Berg et al., 2009). When we are served more food, we eat more food (Sobal & Wansink, 2007). If we are given a big bowl of pretzels, we will eat more than if we are given a small bowl of pretzels. In one study, using larger bowls to serve snacks resulted in an increase of 142 calories when compared with smaller bowls (Wansink & Cheney, 2005). We even eat more if the food is gross. People given larger buckets of 2-week-old stale popcorn ate about 34% more, even though it didn't taste good, compared with people given smaller bags of popcorn (Wansink & Kim, 2004). The problem is that when we eat more because the package or serving is bigger, we don't adjust our intake by eating less later in the day (Ledikwe et al., 2005). We also do not even realize that we have eaten more (Sobal & Wansink, 2007)! This may be because we are terrible at judging portion sizes (Sobal & Wansink, 2007).

We will talk about why portion sizes have increased later on when we discuss industry practices, but suffice it to say that portions are much larger now than they were even 50 years ago. In 1957, the average fast-food hamburger weighed one ounce and the average soda was eight ounces (Nicklas, Baranowski, Cullen, & Berenson, 2001). In 1997, the average burger was six ounces (600% bigger than 40 years ago) and the average soda was between 32 and 64 ounces (800% bigger!). The average-size movie popcorn contained three cups in 1957, compared with 16 cups for a medium-sized popcorn in 1997. Portions in the

United States are 25% bigger than in France, where the prevalence of obesity is much lower (Ledikwe et al., 2005).

Increasing portion sizes would not be a problem if we could regulate how much we eat. But research shows that we respond more to environmental cues than to our own feelings of fullness. A very clever study (Wansink, Painter, & North, 2005) looked at this issue by utilizing "bottomless bowls." Researchers had participants eat soup from either a normal bowl, or from a bowl that would secretly refill itself. Essentially, it was the never-ending bowl of soup. Participants eating from the bottomless bowls ate 73% more than those eating from the normal bowls. What is important here is that the people eating from the bottomless bowls had no idea that they ate more, nor did they feel fuller than those eating from the normal bowls. We use our eyes to determine how much we eat, rather than our stomachs. We eat until the food is gone, rather than eating until we are full (Cohen & Farley, 2008).

We also do not respond to large meals by compensating at the next one through eating less. One scary finding is that whereas children used to be quite adept at balancing their caloric intake throughout a day, children born recently are performing worse and worse at this task. There is a population-wide shift in children's ability to self-regulate their food intake. In the 1980s, children compensated for about 90% of any extra calories they ate in a day (i.e., they would eat less dinner if they had a large snack earlier in the day). By the 1990s, children were only compensating for about 45% of extra calories. It is probably even worse now! The older children get, the worse they are at compensating (Johnson & Taylor-Holloway, 2006).

Soda

Consumption of sodas or sugar-sweetened beverages has increased by 300% over the past several decades (Nielsen & Popkin, 2004). On average, we each now drink around 150 calories per day (Bray, 2010). Sugar-sweetened beverages now contribute more calories to our daily intake than any other food or drink (Woodward-Lopez, Kao, & Ritchie, 2010). Drinking sugar-sweetened beverages, such as soda, is associated with obesity and weight gain among children (Malik, Popkin, Bray, Despres, & Hu, 2010). Although the association is less clear for adults, consuming more soda and/or sugar-sweetened beverages likely contributes to obesity in this group as well (Malik et al., 2010). There are several reasons that sugar-sweetened beverages may contribute to obesity. First, they are empty calories. Sugar-sweetened beverages provide a lot of calories, but don't make people feel full or satisfied (St. Onge et al., 2004). As a result, people don't compensate for calories they drink by adjusting food intake throughout the day (DiMeglio & Mattes, 2000). Second, these beverages are often sweetened with high fructose corn syrup, which some studies suggest contributes to abdominal fat and other health conditions (Bray, 2010; Malik et al., 2010). Soda accounts for more than 40% of the per capita increase in daily calories consumed over the past few decades, and therefore is estimated to be responsible for 20% of the weight gained by the American population since 1977 (Woodward-Lopez, Kao, & Ritchi, 2010).

Interestingly, diet soda does not appear to be a much healthier choice. Although the research is conflicting, some studies have found that consumption of diet soda is associated with obesity and other health problems, such as diabetes (Yantis & Hunter, 2010). This is a bit of a chicken-and-egg problem, however, since it may be that obese or overweight people choose diet soda because they are trying to lose weight. Or it may be that the artificial sweeteners in diet sodas predispose us to sugar cravings and overindulging in other sweets (Yantis & Hunter, 2010). Either way, water is a better choice.

Variety

A larger variety of foods increases intake (Brondel et al., 2009). For example, if you order a very large appetizer sampler, you will eat more than if you ordered the same amount of a single type of appetizer. Or if there are a variety of flavors, we will eat more than if we taste just one flavor. We will eat more French fries if they have ketchup than alone, we will eat more brownies if served with ice cream than without (Brondel et al., 2009). We will eat more of a sandwich with several different fillings than a plain peanut butter one (Sorensen, Moller, Flint, Martens, & Raben, 2003). We will eat more M&M's or jelly beans if we are served a bowl with seven colors than with seven colors (Wansink, 2004). Do you think the manufacturers of these candies are aware of this? When was the last time you saw a bag of all brown M&M's? Variety is the spice of life, and sadly a contributing partner in the obesity epidemic.

There are several reasons that variety may lead us to eat more. When we eat one type of food, we habituate to taste and the palatability of the food decreases as we eat it (Brondel et al., 2009; Sorensen et al., 2003). In other words, the food tastes better on the first bite than on the 25th bite. With a variety of foods, we can have 30 first bites that will taste really good instead of getting bored with one taste. This might explain why people will often not finish their dinner but suddenly have room for dessert (or as some of our family members call it, our second stomach). Another possibility is that it takes us longer to feel full when we eat a bunch of different things as opposed to one thing, so we tend to eat more. Yet another explanation is that we are hardwired to eat many different foods to get enough of the various vitamins and minerals that we need (Cohen, 2008). Regardless of the actual mechanism, it does seem that the food industry has figured out that variety makes us eat more. More than 10,000 new food products are introduced each year (Cohen, 2008).

Meal Patterns and Snacking

Eating breakfast has been associated with lower BMIs in children and adults (Dubois, Girard, Kent, Farmer, & Tatone-Tokuda, 2008). In contrast, eating at night has been associated with obesity (Berg et al., 2009). This may be because people overeat later in the day after skipping breakfast, likely because they are especially hungry and tend to eat quickly, and therefore end up consuming more calories overall. Skipping meals is also associated with obesity (Nicklas et al., 2001), probably for the same reason.

Eating fast is associated with eating more, and vice versa (Andrade, Greene, & Melanson, 2008). If you eat more slowly, you'll probably eat less. This is why your mother may have yelled at you to "stop inhaling your food." It takes time (about 20 minutes) for our stomachs to let our brains know that we are full. When we eat too fast, we can easily eat past the point of capacity before our stomachs have a chance to say, "enough already!" This is the strategy often employed in eating competitions; to eat as quickly as possible at first until the stomach tells the brain to cease and desist.

Another eating pattern that is associated with increased caloric intake is snacking. As a society, we have moved more and more toward constant eating. Restaurants are open until 2:00 am (or sometimes 24 hours) so we can eat in the middle of the night. Drive-throughs allow us to have full meals in our cars. Food is sold in trucks, sold on street corners, and even offered to us for free in the mall to allure us. Food is everywhere, and we eat it everywhere. Even events that should have nothing to do with food have now become opportunities for snacking. Why is it that most bookstores now have a coffee shop within them? What about shopping for books necessitates a large latte and pastry? One of our favorite examples of how absurd American food culture has become is Disney World. Of course, you get the standard popcorn, cotton candy, and soda at Disney. Those are to be expected. But for the truly brave, you can get a dinosaur-size turkey leg to gnaw on while waiting for Space Mountain. What could be more appealing in 90° weather, 10 minutes before riding a roller coaster, than a turkey leg the size of your head?

Although snacking on a giant turkey leg at Disney World or having lattes and pastries at the local bookstore may not be a regular phenomenon, Americans are now snacking more in their everyday lives than they did in the past. Both children and adults snack more now than they did several decades ago, and more frequent snacking has been associated with greater caloric intake and obesity (Piernas & Popkin, 2010a, 2010b). Children consumed about 200 more calories in snacks each day in 2006 than they did in 1977, with higher snacking leading to higher overall caloric intake (Piernas & Popkin, 2010b; U.S. Department of Agriculture, 2010). The problem of huge portion sizes applies to our snacks as well as our meals. We may "snack" from a family-size bag of pretzels while watching TV, and before we know it, the bag is half gone.

There is an important caveat to note with respect to snacking. Snacking can be protective against obesity if it causes us to eat less overall. For example, if we have a light, healthy snack in the afternoon (e.g., carrots, not donuts) and then we eat less at dinner, then our overall caloric intake for the day may be less than if we had not snacked. So snacks are not necessarily evil. In fact, a recent study found that teens who snacked were less likely to be obese than teens who did not snack (Keast, Nicklas, & O'Neill, 2010).

All in all, the research is unclear as to whether snacking is bad or good for our health. Since there have not been any randomized controlled trials of snacking (yet), we cannot say for sure whether snacking increases or decreases the risk of obesity. In the absence of hard science, we could probably safely theorize that certain kinds of snacking (e.g., fruits and vegetables, lean proteins, whole grains) are healthy for us, whereas snacking on cookies and soda is not.

PHYSICAL ACTIVITY

Obviously, there are two sides to the energy equation; one being diet and the other being physical activity. The calories burned in physical activity are an important factor in determining body weight. It is probably common knowledge by now that the more time you spend in sedentary activities (e.g., watching TV, playing video games, sitting at a computer), the higher your weight is likely to be. More physical activity leads to a reduced risk of becoming overweight or obese. Physical activity is also extremely important for people who have lost weight and are trying to keep it off (Fox & Hillsdon, 2007; Haskell et al., 2007). Many researchers have theorized that a trend toward more sedentary lifestyles has in fact contributed to the growing rates of obesity seen in the United States and elsewhere (Fox & Hillsdon, 2007).

Decades ago, many people worked in manual labor jobs, where they were relatively active throughout the day. Today, many of those jobs have been mechanized, leaving people sitting at a desk most of the day as opposed to working the assembly line. Think of all the technologies that have been developed in the past several decades and how they have impacted our activity levels. Computers allow us to have virtually any piece of information available at our fingertips. No longer do we have to make a trip to the library to scour the encyclopedias for the information we need (does anyone even remember having encyclopedias?). Escalators and elevators take the work out of going up stairs, and most people tend to use that option. Remote controls remove the need to get up from the couch to change the channel. Netflix makes a trip to the local video store obsolete. We can even order our groceries online and have them brought to our doorstep, or go to drive-through, allowing us to purchase and receive food without actually having to walk more than a few paces. Sit-down mowers, "moving sidewalks" at the airport, "the Clapper," electronic fishing rods—the list goes on of inventions that reduce physical strain or activity. If you think about it, you could probably meet all your needs and survive for quite some time without ever leaving your couch, or at least your home.

As a society, we have almost completely engineered physical activity out of our daily lives. Some have estimated that we now burn 250 to 500 *fewer* calories per day than we did 50 years ago (Fox & Hillsdon, 2007), which could lead to a difference of more than 50 pounds per year (it takes an imbalance of 3,500 calories to gain or lose one pound)! Research has shown that Americans, on the whole, are failing to meet physical activity recommendations. More than 60% of Americans do not get enough physical activity to see any health benefits, and more than 25% are completely sedentary (Goldberg & King, 2007). You can imagine that these numbers are probably even higher when you consider that some people were not completely honest when self-reporting this information ("Sure, I exercised five days last week…if you count walking to the refrigerator as exercise."). What is the recommended level of activity? According to the American College of Sports Medicine (ACSM) and the American Heart Association, adults should get about 30 minutes of moderate intensity physical activity (e.g., brisk walking), on most (at least 5) days of the week; or 20 minutes of vigorous activity (e.g., jogging) at least 3 days per week; plus 8 to 10 strength-training exercises of 8 to 12 repetitions at least twice per week (Haskell et al., 2007). For weight gain prevention or weight loss, at least 60 to 90 minutes per day of activity are recommended.

Physical activity is important for health, beyond the effect it has on body weight. Being physically active can reduce a person's risk for a number of diseases, such as coronary heart disease, diabetes, some cancers, and even depression (Fox & Hillsdon, 2007; Goldberg & King, 2007). To quell one popular debate, it *is* possible to be physically fit and also overweight or obese. Physical fitness reduces disease risk for those who are overweight or obese, even if it does not result in substantial weight loss (Fox & Hillsdale, 2007).

Television Watching

One behavior that has attracted a lot of attention, particularly with respect to childhood obesity, is TV watching. The more time that children spend watching TV or playing electronic games, the higher their risk of obesity (Fox & Hillsdon, 2007). Unfortunately, children are spending more time in these sedentary activities than ever before. TV is really a triple threat in terms of contributing to obesity. When children watch TV or play video games, less time is spent engaging in calorie expenditure. Second, children are also frequently snacking while in front of the screen. Finally, hours in front of the TV mean hours of exposure to food advertisements, most of which are for unhealthy sugar-laden cereals, sodas, fast food, snacks, or candy (Powell, Szczypka, & Chaloupka, 2007; Powell, Szczypka, Chaloupka, & Braunschweig, 2007). Watching TV while eating increases intake (Stroebele & DeCastro, 2004). We eat more when we are distracted, be it by TV, listening to something or someone, driving, or reading (Wansink, 2004). Obese people have a greater tendency to be distracted and tend to eat more when distracted than nonobese people (Wansink, 2004).

DIET VS. PHYSICAL ACTIVITY: WHICH IS MORE IMPORTANT?

One debate that seems to be very popular in the media is whether obesity is due to lack of physical activity or to poor diet. One week, there will be an "expert" on the local news telling us that lack of exercise is driving the obesity epidemic. The next week there will be a different "expert" saying that the obesity epidemic is due to our proclivity for super-sized, heart-attack-on-a-plate burgers. Of course, representatives of the food industry have their own battalion of "scientists" putting out the message that it is really all about physical activity. Then, you have the diet and weight-loss industry, on the other hand, saying that we should really buy the latest book (or shake, or meal replacement, or some other product) because it will change how we eat so we can keep the weight off *forever! No unpleasant exercise required!* This is typically accompanied by a paragraph of impossibly small text offering some kind of disclaimer such as: "results not typical."

Hopefully by this point it is obvious that both physical activity and diet are important to weight. However, for those of you who are not satisfied by that response and want us to take a stand, here it is: diet is more important. At both the individual level, and the societal level, we give the edge to dietary intake in the battle of importance. We cannot emphasize enough that physical activity is crucial for health. By giving the edge to diet, we are simply saying that what we eat is largely responsible for obesity and will likely be a more effective target of efforts to halt the epidemic. Here is why.

First, at the individual level, it is easy to throw off your energy balance by 100 calories with just few bites of bagel or with one can of soda. On a daily basis, we eat an extra 100 calories in the blink of an eye without even realizing it. We may mindlessly finish off a bag of chips while watching TV (or writing a book), or someone may offer us a piece of chocolate while we wait in front of the microwave at work. How much time and effort does it take to throw off the diet side of the energy balance? Virtually no time. It may take some mental effort if you really want that soda and choose to abstain, but most of the time, we probably overeat without even noticing. No mental effort required. Now, on the physical activity side of the equation, what does it take to throw off your energy balance by 100 calories? You could walk a mile or two, go bowling for 3 hours, or bike for 20 minutes. Clearly, these activities require a lot more time and effort (both physical and mental) to carry out than doing without a few bites of bread. The ACSM recommended that we engage in 45 to 60 minutes of moderate physical activity every day for weight gain prevention. If you are a single mother with two kids and a full-time job, where are you going to find an hour per day to devote to exercise? Forgoing that soda seems like a more realistic alternative at the individual level. (Again, not to condone slacking on physical activity—everyone should strive to meet those ACSM guidelines.)

Second, at the societal level, there is some research to suggest that it is largely changes in our dietary intake that have driven the obesity epidemic (McCrory, Suen, & Roberts, 2002). Some of the increase in obesity can be attributed to declines in energy expenditure, but for the most part, it is the increase in caloric intake that has led to the rising rates of obesity. Overall, it has been estimated that about 93% of the increase in obesity rates across developed nations can be attributed to increases in caloric intake, leaving 7% to be explained by declines in physical activity (Bleich, Cutler, Murray, & Adams, 2008). When it comes to weight, what we eat appears to be driving the bus.

So now that we have answered the diet vs. physical activity debate, we will discuss a variety of other factors that have been associated with obesity. These other factors do not directly influence body weight, but are related to obesity through their effects on either energy intake or expenditure (or both, in some cases). We will start with family and social factors and then progressively broaden our scope to finally look at wide-scale sociocultural, political, and economic factors.

FAMILY AND SOCIAL FACTORS

When was the last time you ate alone? Eating is often a social event. We eat at parties and with others in restaurants. In fact, it's sometimes awkward to spend time with someone without engaging in some activity, and eating is quite common (e.g., "let's grab lunch"). When we celebrate some occasion, we often go out to dinner. Unfortunately, we tend to eat more when we are with others than when alone (Vartanian, Herman, & Polivy, 2007). The larger the group, the more we eat; we eat 76% more calories when in a group of seven or more people than we would if we were alone (Stroebele & deCastro, 2004).

Social constructs such as "meal time" also influence our eating patterns, and therefore our weights. If people think it is time to eat, they will eat, regardless of whether they are hungry or not. People see that it is noon and therefore time for lunch, or they are watching TV so it is time for a snack. Hunger often has nothing to do with it. In a study of people with amnesia, participants ate a complete dinner and were then told 10 to 30 minutes later that it was dinner time. Guess what happened! They ate a second complete meal (Rozin, Dow, Moscovitch, & Rajaram, 1998)!

In terms of families, children emulate the eating behaviors of their parents and siblings, whereas teens tend to also model the eating habits of their peers in addition to their families (Patrick & Nicklas, 2005; Stroebele & De Castro, 2004). Often, children are neophobic about new foods—they refuse to try new things. Offering new foods regularly can overcome children's initial distaste, so it is important for parents to continue to try to expose children to new foods. As few as ten exposures to a food can create a preference (or at least acceptance) of a new food, despite initial wariness (Wardle, Herrera, Cooke, & Gibson, 2003). So, if at first you don't succeed, try, try again. One caveat is that repeated insistence on trying a particular food (as opposed to simply offering it) can actually increase a child's distaste for it, and forbidding certain foods can increase the desire for those foods. In other words, children want to do the opposite of what their parents say (no surprise there!). The more you plead with them to eat their green beans, the less they like the green beans. And if you totally ban them from eating Cocoa Puffs and Reese's Pieces, it only makes them want those items even more. It seems that the best approach is to provide many exposures to a variety of healthier foods and limit exposures to unhealthy items. This authoritative approach to food has been associated with children eating more fruits and vegetables and less junk food (Patrick & Nicklas, 2005). A permissive or authoritarian parenting style of feeding is associated with lower intake of fruits and vegetables and higher body mass (Patrick & Nicklas, 2005).

Some studies have found that frequent family meals and consistent meal patterns are protective against obesity (Nicklas et al., 2001). The effects of having regular family meals are not consistent across gender and age groups, though they do seem to be protective against obesity for younger girls (Fulkerson, Neumark-Sztainer, Hannan, & Story, 2008). This may be because when children eat at home with their families, they are more likely to eat a home-cooked meal as opposed to eating out at a restaurant or fast-food joint where the options are less healthful.

Other family factors also relate to diet and weight. Parent socioeconomic status, employment, and education all influence what kinds of foods are purchased or available in the home, which in turn has an effect on weight (Drewnowski, 2009; Patrick & Nicklas, 2005). Healthy food tends to be more expensive than unhealthy food, so those with lower incomes are less able to afford the healthier alternatives. The next time you are hungry and have only $1.00 in your pocket, walk into a grocery store and compare the prices of a small fruit salad with maybe seven or eight bites of fresh fruit to a packet of prepackaged cupcakes. If you were hungry and had only $1.00, which would you choose?

Individuals and parents who work long hours have little time for food purchasing and preparation, leaving them to rely on convenience or fast food, which tends to be higher in fat, sodium, and calories than food prepared at home. Individuals with higher levels of education may be better able to understand dietary guidelines and advice. They may also put a higher premium on healthy behaviors such as diet and exercise.

COMMUNITY FACTORS

People eat more food if it is more available. If you are at work and there is a bowl of candy on your desk, you will eat more of it than if there is a bowl of candy down the hall on someone else's desk (Wansink, Painter, & Lee, 2006). You will eat more candy if it is in a transparent jar than if it is in an opaque jar. We eat more when food is closer and when we see it all the time (Cohen & Farley, 2008). If you look around your community, whether it be your home, school, or workplace, food is available nearly everywhere. It used to be that food was sold only in certain locations. Eating in your car was unheard of, as was finding a coffee shop in a bookstore, a vending machine on every floor of an office building, or a sandwich shop in a gas station. Pharmacies sold drugs, not groceries and candy. Now, food is ubiquitous.

The types of food stores in our communities have an impact on our weight. People who live in neighborhoods with more supermarkets have a lower risk of obesity, whereas people who live in neighborhoods with more fast-food restaurants and convenience stores tend to have a higher risk of obesity (Story, Kaphingst, Robinson-O'Brien, & Glanz, 2008). If schools are closer to fast-food restaurants, the students in those schools are more likely to be obese than students who go to schools far away from fast-food restaurants (Currie, DellaVigna, Moretti, & Pathania, 2009).

Recall from Chapter 1 that low-income individuals and some racial and ethnic subpopulations are at greater risk for obesity. One explanation for these disparities rests in the fact that food outlets and physical activity spaces are not equitably distributed by neighborhood. For example, poor neighborhoods have about only one third the number of supermarkets as compared with wealthier neighborhoods, but a greater number of fast-food outlets, convenience stores, and alcohol outlets (Morland, Wing, Diez Roux, & Poole, 2002). Within urban areas, predominantly African American neighborhoods have a greater proportion of restaurants categorized as fast-food outlets (as opposed to full service restaurants) than predominantly Caucasian neighborhoods (Powell, Chaloupka, & Bao, 2007).

Not only are there disparities in the types of food outlets that are available in various communities, but also the healthfulness of foods found within grocery stores differ by neighborhood. In Baltimore, for example, one study found a much greater variety and abundance of healthy foods found in grocery stores in predominantly Caucasian, higher-income neighborhoods compared with predominantly low-income or African American neighborhoods (Franco, Diez Roux, Glass, Caballero, & Brancati, 2008). For residents in these latter neighborhoods, even if there is a "grocery store" nearby, the only healthy foods offered may be some bruised bananas or old onions (which typically are also priced much higher than you would find in the average suburban supermarket). One study of parent perceptions of food availability in low-income and predominantly minority areas described stores that sold food that had clearly been eaten by rodents (Sealy, 2010). Understandably, residents are going to be hesitant to buy fresh foods if all that is available to them are some rotten bananas and scraps of potatoes that the rats couldn't finish.

On the physical activity side of the equation, similar disparities are seen in our communities. Low-income and predominantly African American neighborhoods have fewer physical activity facilities than higher-income or primarily Caucasian communities (Gordon-Larsen, Nelson, Page, & Popkin, 2006; Sallis & Glanz, 2006). There are also safety issues with accessing these physical activity spaces (e.g., parks, playgrounds, YMCAs, etc.) when residents may have to travel through crime-ridden areas or walk along streets without sidewalks. There are a variety of neighborhood risks that are not equitably distributed across different populations. These environmental or community factors likely contribute to the disparities we see in obesity rates (and other health issues) across racial and ethnic groups or income levels (Lovasi, Hutson, Guerra, & Neckerman, 2009).

It is difficult to follow any sort of healthy diet if you simply do not have access to healthy foods because they are too expensive or only sold at stores miles and miles away that you cannot travel to because there are no transportation options. It is also difficult to exercise if you do not have access to safe places to be active because they are too far, too expensive, or not safe. Just like you would expect the way our streets are built to have an impact on traffic accidents, the way our communities are built has an impact on our diet and exercise patterns, and therefore our weights.

SOCIOCULTURAL FACTORS

There are several sociocultural factors that have led to higher caloric intake and lower levels of physical activity. Over the past several decades, the United States has seen a larger proportion of women entering the workforce, which has resulted in a heightened demand for convenience foods. As women started working, they had less time for meal preparation and cleanup. In 1900, the average woman spent 44 hours per week on meal preparation and cleanup. In 1975, people spent only 10 hours per week on food preparation (French, Story, & Jeffery, 2001). Likely even less time is spent on food preparation and cleanup now. As we have less and less time to devote to cooking and cleaning, there is a greater demand for convenience and restaurant food.

Additionally, technological advances in food processing and transportation have allowed restaurants to provide a variety of highly tasty foods for less money (Bleich et al., 2008; French et al., 2001). We now have frozen meals, prewashed and cut salads, and prepared foods in the grocery store, as well as fast-food and other quick-service restaurants to choose from for every meal. You could easily get through the rest of your life without actually cooking a single thing. In fact, one of our grandmother's friends has revealed that she has never used her oven in the entire 20-something years she has lived in her apartment. Her oven functions as a storage space for crackers and other snacks! The smoke alarms once went off when someone came to visit and tried to preheat the oven. True story.

Sometimes, we can resist cravings or urges, but many times (particularly when we are stressed, or distracted), we cannot. We only have so much mental energy at any given time to devote to various thoughts or activities. When we use up this mental effort on certain activities, we have less of it to devote to efforts to eat healthfully. We like to refer to this as "cognitive traffic." For example, one group of people was asked to memorize a two-digit number and one group was asked to memorize a seven-digit number. They both were then offered fruit salad or chocolate cake. The people who were asked to memorize the seven-digit number were more likely to choose the chocolate cake (Shiv & Fedorikhin, 1999). Their mental reserves were exhausted by the simple task of memorizing a number, and they had little capacity left to devote to making the healthy choice of fruit. This kind of impulse control and judgment is part of a set of skills often referred to as executive functioning; yet working memory also requires executive functioning from the same part of the brain. In this case, requiring people to heavily tax their working memory skills prevented them from employing impulse control, resulting in reaching for the chocolate cake. If you think about this in the context of our modern and hectic lives, where we often face many competing demands for our attention (e.g., our families, work, school, friends, etc.), it is no wonder that choosing the right foods to eat falls somewhere at the bottom of the list.

In essence, food has become cheaper and more accessible, particularly unhealthy processed and convenience or prepared foods. As unhealthy food has become cheaper and more readily available (and healthy foods are increasingly expensive and more difficult to access), we buy (and eat) more and more junk.

FOOD INDUSTRY PRACTICES

There are many people who espouse the belief that the McDonald's and Burger Kings and Coca-Colas of the world bribed us to overconsume nuggets, fries, and soda by using tiny Disney character toys and cute cartoons to lure us in as children. When put this way, it does sound particularly insidious. However, to be fair (sort of), the food industry is simply doing its job. They are in the business of selling a product, and the more they sell, the more profits they see and the happier their shareholders. So can you really blame them for doing everything they possibly can, including spending millions on advertising and Disney character toy distribution, to boost sales?

The food industry employs various strategies to increase how much and how frequently we eat. Their job is to sell as much food as possible, and they are excellent at it. They use advertising, packaging, variety, lighting, noise levels in restaurants, and even product naming to increase the likelihood that we will purchase more food. For example, detailed menu descriptions such as "succulent shrimp" instead of just shrimp, or "decadent 10-layer ooey-gooey chocolate cake smothered with our signature homemade fudge syrup" instead of just chocolate cake make us want to eat that item more (Wansink, 2004). Listening to music while eating increases intake (Stroebele & DeCastro, 2004). Loud and fast music makes people eat faster and quickens turnover, whereas slow and soft music makes people stay longer in a restaurant. When shelf space for an item doubles in a grocery store, people purchase a lot more of that item, even if the item is unpopular (Cohen & Farley, 2008). Grocery stores also use displays at the ends of aisles and other promotional strategies to increase sales. As a result of all of these industry practices, we buy (and eat) more food. Next time you visit your favorite restaurant or grocery store, look around. You can bet that every detail you see was a deliberate decision made to get you to spend more money, and therefore eat more food. In fact, one of our friends once went to the grocery store to get only two items, and later returned having spent more than $80 and forgot one of the two items. Grocery store 1; shopper 0.

One consistent strategy seen across almost every sector of the food industry is the drive toward larger and larger portions.

Restaurants and food producers have steadily shifted the norm when it comes to portion size. From the food industry stand-point, it costs very little for them to increase the size of meals substantially, and they can charge consumers more. In other words, it costs them pennies to supersize your soda, while you pay an additional 25 cents. For the consumer, the added size represents a good value, since the price per unit is less than for the smaller size (e.g., a liter of Coke costs less per ounce than a 12 ounce can of coke). We are driven to buy these larger por-tions not because we want to consume a pound of French fries in a single sitting, but because the supersized options often are the best economic value (Ledikwe et al., 2005). Essentially, it makes sense for consumers to buy in bulk. From the industry standpoint, it costs very little to add a few more ounces of soda or candy bar (King Size, anyone?), and they can then draw large profits from selling us ever-larger portions. The food producer or restaurant makes a sweet profit, and you feel like you got a sweet deal.

Morgan Spurlock documented the consequences of these mega-portions in his 2004 documentary, *Supersize Me!* Spurlock ate all of his meals at McDonald's for one month, and super-sized whenever they offered. As a result, he gained 25 lbs (in one month!) and faced a variety of other nasty consequences. Perhaps a coincidence, perhaps not, McDonald's did away with its supersize option shortly after the film came out. Other chains have simply renamed their largest portions, but haven't decreased the size at all (Young & Nestle, 2007).

MEDIA AND ADVERTISING

Unfortunately, food advertisements and other cues are every-where. The food industry uses these cues to get us to purchase more food. These cues take the form of various ads and market-ing efforts, the ever-present vending machines, the Starbucks on every street corner, or simply placing a variety of candy bars at the checkout counter so we are tempted to buy one impulsively as we wait in line. If you ask a food industry executive what impact their advertising has on the obesity epidemic, you might hear them say, "Well, we just want people to choose our product over the other million products that are out there. After all, our snicker-choco-sugar-butter-jumbo-cookie can be part of a healthy diet. It is just up to the consumer to make healthy choices overall." The problem is, advertising does much more than simply get us to choose Coke over Pepsi.

When people are shown pictures of food, their brains exhibit a response similar to that seen in addicts when shown their favorite drug. When we see food or pictures of food, our brains secrete dopamine, which creates cravings and drives us to eat (Cohen, 2008). Not only are we driven to eat when we might otherwise not but also exposure to food cues before eating causes us to eat more (Ferriday & Brunstrom, 2008). The response to cues is not specific to the item itself. In other words, seeing or smelling pizza will make us eat more pizza if it is available, but it will also make us eat more sandwiches, cookies, or chicken (Ferriday & Brunstrom, 2008). This means that advertisements for Doritos may make us eat more snacks in general, not just more Doritos.

Food advertising also leads us to choose higher fat and higher calorie foods (French et al., 2001). The most heavily advertised products are the unhealthiest—snacks, convenience foods, and sodas (French et al., 2001; Powell et al., 2007; Powell, Szczypka, et al., 2007). The least advertised foods are the healthy items, such as fruits and vegetables. When was the last time you saw a commercial for broccoli? In fact, a recent study looked at what would happen if you ate only what was advertised on TV. Following a 2,000 calorie a day diet of advertised food products would lead you to consume 25 times the recommended amount of sugars, 20 times the recommended amount of fat, and only 40% of the recommended amount of vegetables and 27% of the recommended amount of fruits (Mink, Evans, Moore, Calderon, & Deger, 2010).

Advertising is particularly critical in the case of children, who are too young to even understand that commercials are designed to sell them something. In one study of the effects of ads on children, researchers had children taste food and drinks that were identical except for one set had McDonald's packaging while the other set was unmarked. Children preferred the food and drinks with the McDonalds packaging, indicating that advertising and branding had an impact (Robinson, Borzekowski, Matheson, & Kraemer, 2007). Of course, the food companies know this—that's why they spend so much on marketing their products to us! Because it works! If a friend walked in to your house with two bags of burgers, one in a plain brown bag and one in a bag covered with all your favorite McDonald's characters, which would you go for?

The pervasiveness of food advertising is important because we eat in response to cues or stimuli that surround us, much like an alcoholic responds to a beer advertisement by craving a drink. Our brains are primed to respond to these cues over time by eating, and eating a lot. David Kessler, the former commissioner of the Food and Drug Administration, believes that obese people are more likely to be hypersensitive to these environmental cues and are therefore more likely to eat greater amounts throughout the day, eat past the point of fullness, and to work harder to obtain food (or pay more). Food is simply more reinforcing to obese individuals. Kessler has even coined a term for the "addictiveness" of food: "conditioned hypereating" (p. 145). For a discussion of the addictiveness of food, see Box 2.3. Conditioned hypereating refers to the notion that eating behavior has become automated, and is highly influenced by our environments and the food industries that shape them. Importantly, Kessler says we should not consider conditioned hypereating abnormal or pathological. It is a "psychological adaptation to the environment that occurs among certain susceptible individuals" (p. 162).

BOX 2.3 AM I REALLY ADDICTED TO CHOCOLATE?

Food has long been described in terms we typically associate with addiction. People talk about being "chocoholics," or having cravings for certain foods (pickles and ice cream, anyone?), or being on a "sugar high," or "crashing" after a candy binge. You can probably find meetings for *Food Addicts Anonymous* or *Overeaters Anonymous* in your hometown, if you are so inclined. While food addiction has not yet made it into the Diagnostic and Statistical Manual of Mental Disorders—Fourth Edition (American Psychiatric Association, 2000), there is some evidence that people can show addiction-like behaviors and characteristics in the context of food (especially foods that are high in fat and sugar). Both food and drugs can trigger the release of dopamine, and in studies of brain activity patterns, food cues have been found to cause similar patterns to that of drugs—it activates our brain's reward circuitry (Gearhardt et al., 2011). Certainly, behaviors surrounding food intake can mirror those of substance use: using the "substance" in larger amounts or for a period longer than intended (who hasn't eaten more ice cream than originally planned?), experiencing a persistent desire for the "substance," being unable to limit or reduce use (i.e., failing to follow a diet plan), spending a lot of time seeking or consuming the "substance," and continuing to use the "substance" despite negative consequences (i.e., continuing to eat a diet of fried foods after being diagnosed with high cholesterol; Corwin & Grigson, 2009). Many people report feeling out of control when it comes to particular foods, another key characteristic of substance dependence. All in all, the research is ongoing, but it does seem that there might be some legitimacy to the term "chocoholic."

Another consequence of food marketing is what we like to call "too much information syndrome." In the past week, you have probably seen hundreds of different ads and product labels all telling you that you should buy a particular product because it has vitamin C or lots of fiber, or is low-carb, or it will help your immunity, and so on. There are thousands upon thousands of products being hawked at us, and we are given as many reasons to choose one product over the other. One consequence of having this information overload is that we end up making poor decisions when it comes to our health. When people are presented with too much information, they can't process all of it, and end up making a choice that requires as little mental effort as possible (Cohen, 2008). We operate on impulse, or go with a default choice. So instead of choosing the grilled-chicken and tomato sandwich (because tomatoes have lycopene!) or the low-carb omelet (because carbs go straight to your waistline!), we get overwhelmed by all of the information presented and err toward our old standby, the cheeseburger, which is usually cheaper anyway.

GEOGRAPHIC FACTORS

As we discussed above when we talked about food availability, where we live (and work and play) has an impact on our weight. Within the United States, there are regional differences in rates of obesity. States in the South tend to have higher rates of obesity than states in the North or Midwest (Centers for Disease Control and Prevention, 2010; Ezzati, Martin, Skjold, Vander Hoorn, & Murray, 2006; Tudor-Locke, Kronenfeld, Kim, Benin, & Kuby, 2007). There are various cultural differences in the way we eat, work, and play that are dependent upon where we are from or where we live in the United States. For example, "Southern Cooking" refers to a pattern of high-fat cooking, often including fried foods. If you have ever lived in the South, you may have seen things such as fried pickles or fried okra. These items are not often seen on menus in other parts of the country. Of course, high-fat and high-calorie foods can be found everywhere. However, there are clearly cultural or regional patterns in our diets that vary across geographic areas.

In fact, the Southeastern region of the country is referred to as the "stroke belt" because of the particularly high incidence of stroke across these states, which include Alabama, Arkansas, Georgia, Indiana, Kentucky, Louisiana, Mississippi, North and South Carolina, Tennessee, and Virginia (Barker, Kirtland, Gregg, Geiss, & Thompson, 2011; Hajjar & Kotchen, 2003). Residents in these states tend to eat a diet higher in sodium than other Americans (Hajjar & Kotchen, 2003). Recently, a "diabetes belt" has also been identified across a similar area of the United States, with the addition of portions of Florida, Ohio, Pennsylvania, Texas, and West Virginia (Barker et al., 2011). You also see differences in physical activity. People living in the "diabetes belt" tend to be more sedentary, and more likely to be obese than those who live elsewhere in the United States (Barker et al., 2011).

Rural and urban areas tend to have higher rates of obesity than suburban areas (Nelson, Gordon-Larsen, Song, & Popkin, 2006), which likely reflects a lot of the community-level factors we described above. Residents of both rural and urban areas typically have lower incomes than residents of suburban areas. People who live in rural areas may have to travel long distances to get their groceries, and may have few options available to them in terms of food stores and physical activity spaces. People in low-income urban areas likely have many more options immediately available, but they may not be healthy options, and residents may not have cars or transportation to get to a supermarket. People in suburbia, by contrast, will most likely have access to parks and at least one car, making it easier for them to get to a supermarket or physical activity facility. Supermarkets tend to locate themselves in the suburbs as well, since property is cheaper and they can have large parking lots (a virtual impossibility in an urban city center).

FOOD PRICE AND SOCIOECONOMIC FACTORS

A basic tenet of economics is that as price goes down, demand goes up. If the price of candy bars declines, more candy bars will be purchased. Since the 1970s, the relative price of food (compared with other things we buy) has been falling. Food prices have decreased by 38% overall since 1978 (Council of Economic Advisors, 2005). This might be all well and good if the prices of healthy foods had dropped as much as (or more than) the prices of unhealthy foods. However, as you might have surmised, the prices of unhealthy foods (e.g., calorie-dense, low-nutrient, high-fat, and sugar foods) have fallen drastically, whereas the price of fresh fruits and vegetables has increased by 190% since the early 1980s (Drewnowski & Darmon, 2005; Finkelstein & Strombotne, 2010). We will discuss the price of foods later in this chapter. Given these price differentials, it is no wonder that our intake of unhealthy, calorie-dense food has skyrocketed, whereas our intake of fruits and vegetables is, in relative terms, abysmal.

Another cost that we often don't think of is the time it costs us to acquire and prepare food. Our grandparents spent hours and hours every week buying, preparing, and cooking food. We merely have to pull over to the drive-through for a five-minute detour, or buy completely pre-prepared meals from the grocery store. Think about how one invention—the microwave—has drastically reduced our food preparation times. It is simply a lot easier than it used to be to put food in our mouths.

A third cost you might not have considered in the context of obesity is the cost of actually being overweight or obese. Because we now have cholesterol-lowering pills or blood-pressure medication available, the consequences of being obese are not felt in the same way they were decades ago. Typically, these medications are covered by our health insurance, so we likely do not even realize the true cost of dealing with these health issues.

AGRICULTURAL POLICY

To understand why some foods are more expensive than others, we have to look where our food comes from and how it is produced. Agricultural policy has historically focused on ensuring that there is enough food to adequately feed our country. Though hunger has been and continues to be, a major problem, we now produce more than enough food to go around. The U.S. food supply provides almost 4,000 calories per person per day. This has increased by about 700 calories per person per day since the early 1980s (Young & Nestle, 2007). Some of these extra calories are lost through food spoilage and waste, but even after taking that into account, there is still an overabundance of calories being produced. Food oversupply is now more of a problem than food shortage (at least in the United States). What's more is that certain foods are overproduced, while there is a shortage of other foods (such as fruits and vegetables). For example, there are not enough fruits and vegetables being produced for every American to meet dietary guidelines. U.S. production of fruit would need to increase by 117% and vegetable production by 135% to have an adequate supply (Buzby, Wells, & Vocke, 2006).

Agriculture looked very different 100 years ago than it does today. Whereas there used to be a plethora of small- and medium-sized farms across the United States, food production is now very concentrated among a handful of industry titans. In essence, agriculture went from providing a service at a local level (producing food for Americans) to becoming a money-making global enterprise (like the banking and pharmaceutical industries). There was a huge level of consolidation and vertical integration. Vertical integration refers to a few companies taking over the entire spectrum of food production activities. Whereas there used to be separate entities responsible for farming, processing, shipping, and packaging, vertical integration allowed one large company to own and control all of those components. The result of these changes was an increase in productivity—more food for less!

At the same time, government policies facilitated this transition and provided a variety of incentives that shaped our current food system. The federal government started paying farmers in the early 20th century to produce certain crops in order to maintain a stable supply of these staples. In the 1970s, as agriculture became a global economic enterprise, these payments (referred to as farm subsidies) served to boost production of items that could be sold on international markets. The most highly subsidized crops are corn, wheat, soybeans, rice, barley, oats, and sorghum (Jackson, Minjares, Naumoff, Shrimali, & Martin, 2009). The effect of subsidizing these crops is that farms (large and small) shift to produce these items at the exclusion of others, such as fruits and vegetables. We then are left with tons of corn, wheat, and soybeans, and not enough fruits and vegetables.

As supply goes up, price comes down. While the price of calorie-dense foods increased by 20% to 46% between 1985 and 2000, the price of fresh fruits and vegetables increased by 118% (Drewnowski & Darmon, 2005; Finkelstein & Strombotne, 2010). Obviously, food processors and other operations want to use the cheapest ingredients. So instead of using sugar to sweeten soda, companies switched to high-fructose corn syrup because it was so much cheaper (and abundant). Instead of gasoline, we now have cars that run partly on corn ethanol. Instead of feeding their cattle with grass, beef producers started to force feed their cows corn and soybeans. Cheap animal feed translates to cheaper meat; which is in part why we can now get a hamburger for 99 cents. Another consequence of the oversupply of certain food items was that the food industry had to invent ways to get us to eat more; hence, the industry practices we described above, such as bigger portion sizes, increasing availability, and heavy marketing efforts.

Lest you think that the American farmer is sitting there getting rich off of subsidy payments (some of them are, but most are not), the real winner in American agricultural policy is the large food processing companies. There are a handful of mega-corporations that are responsible for the vast majority of food production in the United States. These companies buy the cheapest ingredients they can from farmers, who are often forced to accept rock-bottom prices for their crops. The food processing companies can then create thousands of tasty processed foods and charge consumers a huge markup (and make huge profits). In 1980, farmers received 31 cents of every food dollar spent; in 2000, they received only 19 cents (Jackson et al., 2009). The other 81 cents went to the food producers, who spend that money on things such as packaging, research and development, transportation, and marketing.

What does all this have to do with obesity? Well, for one, agriculture policy and the industrialization of our food supply has made processed and convenience foods extremely cheap, yet widely available. At the same time, fruits and vegetables are in short supply and have increased in price over time. In essence, we (well, our government and the forces that influence it) have created a food system that encourages us to eat poorly and too much.

In Sum

We have covered the major of the causes of obesity, but there are far too many to even list in a book chapter, let alone describe in any depth. Hopefully, what you take away from this chapter is that obesity is a very complex problem, with a huge web of causal factors. Some of these determinants are more important than others, but the obesity epidemic is obviously not going to be an easy one to fix.

NOTES

[1]See Box 1.1 for a description of correlations.
[2]See Box 2.1 for a primer in genetic terminology.
[3]Interestingly, this is why crash diets are often unsustainable. Someone may starve himself or herself and lose 30 pounds in a short period of time, but because they have trained their body to save as much energy as possible, they easily put on weight when they return to a normal diet.

REFERENCES

Agras, W. S., & Mascola, A. J. (2005). Risk factors for childhood overweight. *Current Opinion in Pediatrics, 17*, 648–652.

American Psychiatric Association. (2000). *Diagnostic and statistical manual of mental disorders* (4th ed.-rev.). Washington, DC: Author.

Andrade, A. M., Greene, G. W., & Melanson, K. J. (2008). Eating slowly led to decreases in energy intake within meals in healthy women. *Journal of the American Dietetic Association, 108*, 1186–1191.

Baird, J., Fisher, D., Lucas, P., Kleijnen, J., Roberts, H., & Law, C. (2005). Being big or growing fast: Systematic review of size and growth in infancy and later obesity. *British Medical Journal, 331*, 929–931.

Barcenas, C. H., Wilkinson, A. V., Strom, S. S., Cao, Y., Saunders, K. C., Mahabir, S., . . . Bondy, M. L. (2007). Birthplace, years of residence in the United States, and obesity among Mexican-American adults. *Obesity (Silver Spring, Md.), 15*(4), 1043–1052.

Barker, L. E., Kirtland, K. A., Gregg, E. W., Geiss, L. S., & Thompson, T. J. (2011). Geographic distribution of diagnosed diabetes in the U.S.: A diabetes belt. *American Journal of Preventive Medicine, 40*(4), 434–439.

Bates, L. M., Acevedo-Garcia, D., Alegria, M., & Krieger, N. (2006). Immigration and generational trends in Body Mass Index and obesity in the United States: Results of the National Latino and Asian American Survey, 2002–2003. *American Journal of Public Health, 97,* 70–77.

Bell, J. F., & Zimmerman, F. J. (2010). Shortened nighttime sleep duration in early childhood and subsequent childhood obesity. *Archives of Pediatric and Adolescent Medicine, 164,* 840–848.

Bellisari, A. (2008). Evolutionary origins of obesity. *Obesity Reviews, 9,* 165–180.

Berg, C., Lappas, G., Wolk, A., Strandhagen, E., Torén, K., Rosengren, A., . . . Lissner, L. (2009). Eating patterns and portion size associated with obesity in a Swedish population. *Appetite, 52*(1), 21–26.

Bethell, C., Simpson, L., Stumbo, S., Carle, A. C., & Gombojav, N. (2010). National, state and local disparities in childhood obesity. *Health Affairs, 29,* 347–356.

Bleich, S. N., Cutler, D., Murray, C., & Adams, A. (2008). Why is the developed world obese? *Annual Reviews of Public Health, 29,* 273–295.

Bluher, M. (2009). Adipose tissue dysfunction in obesity. *Experiments in Clinical Endocrinology and Diabetes, 117,* 241–250.

Booth, F. W., & Shanely, R. A. (2004). The biochemical basis of the health effects of exercise: An integrative view. *Proceedings of the Nutrition Society, 63,* 199–203.

Bowman, S. A., Gortmaker, S. L., Ebbeling, C. B., Pereira, M. A., & Ludwig, D. S. (2004). Effects of fast-food consumption on energy intake and diet quality among children in a national household survey. *Pediatrics, 113,* 112–118.

Bray, G. A. (2010). Soft drink consumption and obesity: It is all about fructose. *Current Opinions in Lipidology, 21,* 51–57.

Brondel, L., Romer, M., Van Wymelbeke, V., Pineau, N., Jiang, T., Hanus, C., & Rigaud, D. (2009). Variety enhances food intake in humans: Role of sensory-specific satiety. *Physiology & Behavior, 97*(1), 44–51.

Brown, W. J., Williams, L., Ford, J. H., Ball, K., & Dobson, A. J. (2005). Identifying the energy gap: Magnitude and determinants of 5-year weight gain in mid-age women. *Obesity Research, 13,* 1431–1441.

Brownell, K. D. (2004). Fast food and obesity in children. *Pediatrics, 113,* 132–132.

Buchholz, A. C., & Schoeller, D. A. (2004). Is a calorie a calorie? *American Journal of Clinical Nutrition, 79*(Suppl.), 899S–906S.

Bulik, C. M., Sullivan, P. F., & Kendler, K. S. (2003). Genetic and environmental contributions to obesity and binge eating. *International Journal of Eating Disorders, 33*, 293–298.

Butte, N. F., & Ellis, K. J. (2003). Comment on "obesity and the environment: Where do we go from here?". *Science, 301*, 598b.

Buzby, J. C., Wells, H. F., & Vocke, G. (2006). *Possible implications for U.S. agriculture from adoption of select dietary guidelines* (Economic Research Report No. ERR-31). Washington, DC. Retrieved from http://www.ers.usda.gov/Publications/ERR31/

Campion, J., Milagro, F. I., & Martinez, J. A. (2009). Individuality and epigenetics in obesity. *Obesity Reviews, 10*, 383–392.

Centers for Disease Control and Prevention. (2010). Vital signs: State-specific obesity prevalence among adults—United States, 2009. *Morbidity and Mortality Weekly Report, 59*(30), 950–955.

Chakravarthy, M. V., & Booth, F. W. (2004). Eating, exercise, and "thrifty" genotypes: Connecting the dots toward an evolutionary understanding of modern chronic diseases. *Journal of Applied Physiology, 96*, 3–10.

Chou, S. Y., Grossman, M., & Saffer, H. (2004). An economic analysis of adult obesity: Results from the Behavioral Risk Factor Surveillance System. *Journal of Health Economics, 23*, 565–587.

Christodoulides, C., Scarda, A., Granzotto, M., Milan, G., Dalla Nora, E., Keogh, J.,...Vettor, R. (2006). WNT10B mutations in human obesity. *Diabetologia, 49*(4), 678–684.

Cinti, S. (2005). The adipose organ. *Prostaglandins, Leukotrienes and Essential Fatty Acids, 73*, 9–15.

Clement, K. (2005). Genetics of human obesity. *Proceedings of the Nutrition Society, 64*, 133–142.

Cohen, D. A. (2008). Neurophysiological pathways to obesity: Below awareness and beyond individual control. *Diabetes, 57*, 1768–1773.

Cohen, D. A., & Farley, T. A. (2008). Eating as an automatic behavior. *Preventing Chronic Disease, 5*, 1–7.

Colapinto, C. K., Fitzgerald, A., Taper, L. J., & Veugelers, P. J. (2007). Children's preference for large portions: Prevalence, determinants, and consequences. *Journal of the American Dietetic Association, 107*(7), 1183–1190.

Coppack, S. W. (2005). Adipose tissue changes in obesity. *Biochemical Society Transactions, 33*(5), 1049–1052.

Corwin, R. L., & Grigson, P. S. (2009). Symposium overview—Food addiction fact or fiction? *Journal of Nutrition, 139*, 617–619.

Coughlin, C. C., Halpin, J. V., Magkos, F., Mohammed, B. S., & Klein, S. (2007). Effect of marked weight loss on adiponectin gene expression and plasma concentrations. *Obesity, 15*, 640–645.

Council of Economic Advisors. (2005). *Economic Report of the President, 2005.* Washington, DC: U.S. Government Printing Office. Retrieved from http://a257.g.akamaitech.net/7/257/2422/17feb20051700/www.gpoaccess. gov/eop/2005/2005_erp.pdf

Crowley, V. E. F. (2008). Overview of human obesity and central mechanisms regulating energy homeostasis. *Annals of Clinical Biochemistry, 45*, 245–255.

Cummings, D. E., & Schwartz, M. W. (2003). Genetics and pathophysiology of human obesity. *Annual Reviews in Medicine, 54*, 453–471.

Currie, J., DellaVigna, S., Moretti, E., & Pathania, V. (2009). *The effect of fast food restaurants on obesity* (National Bureau of Economic Research Working Paper Series No. 14721). Washington, DC. Retrieved from http://www.nber.org/papers/w14721

De Castro, J. M. (2004). Genes, the environment and the control of food intake. *British Journal of Nutrition, 92*(Suppl.), S59–S62.

DiMeglio, D. P., & Mattes, R. D. (2000). Liquid versus solid carbohydrate: Effects on food intake and body weight. *International Journal of Obesity and Related Metabolic Disorders, 24*(6), 794–800.

Drewnowski, A. (2009). Obesity, diets, and social inequalities. *Nutrition Reviews, 67*, S36–S39.

Drewnoski, A., & Darmon, N. (2005). Food choices and diet costs: An economic analysis. *American Society of Nutrition Science, 135*, 900–904.

Drolet, R., Richard, C., Sniderman, A. D., Mailloux, J., Fortier, M., Huot, C.,...Tchernof, A. (2008). Hypertrophy and hyperplasia of abdominal adipose tissues in women. *International Journal of Obesity, 32*(2), 283–291.

Dubois, L., Girard, M., Kent, M. P., Farmer, A., & Tatone-Tokuda, F. (2008). Breakfast skipping is associated with differences in meal patterns, macronutrient intakes and overweight among pre-school children. *Public Health Nutrition, 12*, 19–28.

Ebbeling, C. B., Sinclair, K. B., Pereira, M. A., Garcia-Lago, E., Feldman, H. A., & Ludwig, D. S. (2004). Compensation for energy intake from fast food among overweight and lean adolescents. *Journal of the American Medical Association, 291*(23), 2828–2833.

Elder, S. J., Neale, M. C., Das, S., Fuss, P. J., McCrory, M. A., Heymsfield, S. B., … Roberts, S. (2008). Effect of body composition methodology on estimates of fat mass heritability. *Obesity, 16*(S1), S256.

Etelson, D., Brand, D. A., Patrick, P. A., & Shirali, A. (2003). Childhood obesity: Do parents recognize this health risk? *Obesity Research, 11*, 1362–1368.

Ezzati, M., Martin, H., Skjold, S., Vander Hoorn, S., & Murray, C. J. (2006). Trends in national and state-level obesity in the USA after correction for self-report bias: Analysis of health surveys. *Journal of the Royal Society of Medicine, 99*(5), 250–257.

Farooqi, I. S., & O'Rahilly, S. (2007). Genetic factors in human obesity. *Obesity Reviews, 8*(Suppl. 1), 37–40.

Faust, I. M., Johnson, P. R., Stern, J. S., & Hirsh, J. (1978). Diet-induced adipocyte number increase in adult rats: A new model of obesity. *American Journal of Physiology, 235*, 279–286.

Ferriday, D., & Brunstrom, J. M. (2008). How does food-cue exposure lead to larger meal sizes. *British Journal of Nutrition, 100*, 1325–1332.

Field, A. E., Cook, N. R., & Gillman, M. W. (2005). Weight status in childhood as a predictor of becoming overweight or hypertensive in early adulthood. *Obesity Research, 13*, 163–169.

Finkelstein, E. A., & Strombotne, K. L. (2010). The economics of obesity. *American Journal of Clinical Nutrition, 91*(Suppl.), 1520S–1524S.

Fox, F. W. (1973). The enigma of obesity. *Lancet, 2*, 1487–1488.

Fox, K. R., & Hillsdon, M. (2007). Physical activity and obesity. *Obesity Reviews, 8*(Suppl. 1), 115–121.

Franco, M., Diez Roux, A. V., Glass, T. A., Caballero, B., & Brancati, F. L. (2008). Neighborhood characteristics and availability of healthy foods in Baltimore. *American Journal of Preventive Medicine, 35*(6), 561–567.

Frayling, T. M., Timpson, N. J., Weedon, M. N., Zeggini, E., Freathy, R. M., Lindgren, C. M., … McCarthy, M. I. (2007). A common variant in the FTO gene is associated with body mass index and predisposes to childhood and adult obesity. *Science (New York, N.Y.), 316*(5826), 889–894.

Frazao, E. (1999). *America's eating habits: Changes and consequences* (Agriculture Information Bulletin No. AIB750). US Department of Agriculture Economic Research Service. Washington, DC. Retrieved from http://www.ers.usda.gov/Publications/AIB750/

French, S. A., Story, M., & Jeffery, R. W. (2001). Environmental influences on eating and physical activity. *Annual Reviews in Public Health, 22,* 309–335.

French, S. A., Story, M., Neumark-Sztainer, D., Fulkerson, J. A., & Hannan, P. (2001). Fast food restaurant use among adolescents: Associations with nutrient intake, food choices and behavioral and psychosocial variables. *International Journal of Obesity, 25,* 1823–1833.

Fruhbeck, G. (2008). Overview of adipose tissue and its role in obesity and metabolic disorders. *Methods in Molecular Biology, 456,* 1–22.

Fulkerson, J. A., Neumark-Sztainer, D., Hannan, P. J., & Story, M. (2008). Family meal frequency and weight status among adolescents: Cross-sectional and 5-year longitudinal associations. *Obesity, 16,* 2529–2534.

Gardner, D. S., & Rhodes, P. (2009). Developmental origins of obesity: Programming of food intake or physical activity? In B. Koletzko, T. Decsi, D. Molnar, & A. de la Hunty (Eds.), *Early nutrition programming and health outcomes in later life: Obesity and beyond.* New York: Springer Science and Business Media.

Gillman, M. W., Rifas-Shiman, S., Berkey, C. S., Field, A. E., & Colditz, G. A. (2003). Maternal gestational diabetes, birth weight, and adolescent obesity. *Pediatrics, 111,* e221–e226.

Gluckman, P. D., & Hanson, M. A. (2008). Developmental and epigenetic pathways to obesity: An evolutionary-developmental perspective. *International Journal of Obesity, 32,* S62–S71.

Goldberg, J. H., & King, A. C. (2007). Physical activity and weight management across the lifespan. *Annual Reviews of Public Health, 28,* 145–170.

Gordon-Larsen, P., Nelson, M. C., Page, P., & Popkin, B. M. (2006). Inequality in the built environment underlies key health disparities in physical activity and obesity. *Pediatrics, 117,* 417–424.

Guo, S. S., Wu, W., Chumlea, W. C., & Roche, A. F. (2002). Predicting overweight and obesity in adulthood from body mass index values in childhood and adolescence. *American Journal of Clinical Nutrition, 76,* 653–658.

Hajjar, I., & Kotchen, T. (2003). Regional variations of blood pressure in the United States are associated with regional variation in dietary intakes: The NHANES-III data. *The American Society for Nutritional Sciences Journal, 133,* 211–214.

Hales, C. N., & Barker, D. J. (1992). Type 2 (non-insulin-dependent) diabetes mellitus: The thrifty phenotype hypothesis. *Diabetologia, 35,* 595–601.

Harder, T., Bergmann, R., Kallischnigg, G., & Plagemann, A. (2005). Duration of breastfeeding and risk of overweight: A meta-analysis. *American Journal of Epidemiology, 162,* 397–403.

Harrington, J. W., Nguyen, V. Q., Paulson, J. F., Garland, R., Pasquinelli, L., & Lewis, D. (2010). Identifying the "tipping point" age for overweight pediatric patients. *Pediatrics, 49*(7), 638.

Haskell, W. L., Lee, I. M., Pate, R. R., Powell, K. E., Blair, S. N., Franklin, B. A.,...Bauman, A. (2007). Physical activity and public health: Updated recommendation for adults from the American College of Sports Medicine and the American Heart Association. *Medicine and Science in Sports and Exercise, 39*(8), 1423–1434.

Haworth, C. M., Plomin, R., Carnell, S., & Wardle, J. (2008). Childhood obesity: Genetic and environmental overlap with normal-range BMI. *Obesity, 16,* 1585–1590.

He, M., & Evans, A. (2007). Are parents aware that their children are overweight or obese? Do they care? *Canadian Family Physician, 53,* 1493–1499.

Hebebrand, J., & Hinney, A. (2009). Environmental and genetic risk factors in obesity. *Child and Adolescent Psychiatric Clinics of North America, 18,* 83–94.

Herbert, A., Gerry, N. P., McQueen, M. B., Heid, I. M., Pfeufer, A., Illig, T.,...Christman, M. F. (2006). A common genetic variant is associated with adult and childhood obesity. *Science (New York, N.Y.), 312*(5771), 279–283.

Hill, J. O., Wyatt, H. R., Reed, G. W., & Peters, J. C. (2003). Obesity and the environment: Where do we go from here? *Science, 299*(5608), 853–855.

Hjelmborg, J. B., Fagnani, C., Silventoinen, K., McGue, M., Korkeila, M., Christensen, K.,...Kaprio, J. (2008). Genetic influences on growth traits of BMI: A longitudinal study of adult twins. *Obesity (Silver Spring, Md.), 16*(4), 847–852.

Hossain, P., Kawar, B., & El Nahas, M. (2007). Obesity and diabetes in the developing world. *New England Journal of Medicine, 356*, 213–215.

Jackson, R. J., Minjares, R., Naumoff, K. S., Shrimali, B. P., & Martin, L. K. (2009). Agriculture policy is health policy. *Journal of Hunger and Environmental Nutrition, 4*(3), 393–408.

Janssen, I., Katzmarzyk, P. T., Boyce, W. F., Vereecken, C., Mulvihill, C., Roberts, C., ... Pickett, W. (2005). Comparison of overweight and obesity prevalence in school-aged youth from 34 countries and their relationships with physical activity and dietary patterns. *Obesity Reviews, 6*(2), 123–132.

Jo, J., Gavrilova, O., Pack, S., Jou, W., Mullen, S., Sumner, A. E., ... Periwal, V. (2009). Hypertrophy and/or hyperplasia: Dynamics of adipose tissue growth. *Plos Computational Biology, 5*(3), e1000324.

Johnson, S. L., & Taylor-Holloway, L. A. (2006). Non-Hispanic white and Hispanic elementary school children's self-regulation of energy intake. *American Journal of Clinical Nutrition, 83*(6), 1276–1282.

Kaplan, M. S., Huguet, N., Newsom, J. T., & McFarland, B. H. (2004). The association between length of residence and obesity among Hispanic immigrants. *American Journal of Preventive Medicine, 27*(4), 323–326.

Keast, D. R., Nicklas, T. A., & O'Neill, C. E. (2010). Snacking is associated with reduced risk of overweight and reduced abdominal obesity in adolescents: National Health and Nutrition Examination Survey (NHANES) 1999–2004. *American Journal of Clinical Nutrition, 92*(2), 428–435.

Kelly, T., Yang, W., Chen, C. S., Reynolds, K., & He, J. (2008). Global burden of obesity in 2005 and projections to 2030. *International Journal of Obesity, 32*, 1431–1437.

Kessler, D. A. (2009). *The end of overeating: Taking control of the insatiable American appetite.* New York: Rodale Inc.

Koplan, J. P., Liverman, C. T., & Kraak, V. I. (2005). Preventing childhood obesity: Health in the balance: Executive summary. *Journal of the American Dietetic Association, 105*, 131–138.

Landsberg, L., Young, J. B., Leonard, W. R., Linsenmeier, R. A., & Turek, F. W. (2009). Is obesity associated with lower body temperatures? Core temperature: A forgotten variable in energy balance. *Metabolism, 58*(6), 871–876.

Ledikwe, J. H., Ello-Martin, J. A., & Rolls, B. J. (2005). Portion sizes and the obesity epidemic. *Journal of Nutrition, 135*(4), 905–909.

Levin, B. E. (2009). Synergy of nature and nurture in the development of childhood obesity. *International Journal of Obesity, 33*, S53–S56.

Lin, B. H., Guthrie, J., & Frazao, E. (1999). Nutrient contribution of food away from home. In E. Frazao (Ed.), *America's eating habits: Changes and consequences* (pp. 213–242). Washington, DC: US Department of Agriculture and US Economic Research Service.

Loos R. J., & Bouchard, C. (2003). Obesity: Is it a genetic disorder? *Journal of Internal Medicine, 254*(5), 401–425.

Loos, R. J., Rankinen, T., Tremblay, A., Perusse, L., Chagnon, Y., & Bouchard. C. (2005). Melanocortin-4 receptor gene and physical activity in the Quebec Family Study. *International Journal of Obesity, 29*(4), 420–428.

Loos, R. J., Ruchat, S., Rankinen, T., Tremblay, A., Perusse, L., & Bouchard, C. (2007). Adiponectin and adiponectin receptor gene variants in relation to resting metabolic rate, respiratory quotient, and adiposity-related phenotypes in the Quebec Family Study. *American Journal of Clinical Nutrition, 85*, 26–34.

Lovasi, G. S., Hutson, M. A., Guerra, M., & Neckerman, K. M. (2009). Built environments and obesity in disadvantaged populations. *Epidemiological Reviews, 31*, 7–20.

Malik, V. S., Popkin, B. M., Bray, G. A., Despres, J. P., & Hu, F. B. (2010). Sugar-sweetened beverages, obesity, type 2 diabetes mellitus, and cardiovascular disease risk. *Circulation, 121*, 1356–1364.

Malis, C., Rasmussen, E. L., Poulsen, P., Petersen, I., Christensen, K., Beck-Nielsen, H.,...Vaag, A. A. (2005). Total and regional fat distribution is strongly influenced by genetic factors in young and elderly twins. *Obesity Research, 13*(12), 2139–2145.

Martorell, R., Stein, A. D., & Schroeder, D. G. (2001). Early nutrition and later adiposity. *Journal of Nutrition, 131*, 874S–880S.

Massiera, F., Barbry, P., Guesnet, P., Joly, A., Luquet, S., Moreilhon-Brest, C.,...Ailhaud, G. (2010). A Western-like fat diet is sufficient to induce a gradual enhancement in fat mass over generations. *Journal of Lipid Research, 51*(8), 2352–2361.

McCrory, M. A., Suen, V. M., & Roberts, S. B. (2002). Biobehavioral influences on energy intake and adult weight gain. *Journal of Nutrition, 132*, 3830S–3834S.

McPherson, R. (2007). Genetic contributors to obesity. *Canadian Journal of Cardiology, 23* (Suppl. A), 23A–27A.

Melanson, E. L., Astrup, A., & Donahoo, W. T. (2009). The relationship between dietary fat and fatty acid intake and body weight, diabetes, and the metabolic syndrome. *Annals of Nutrition and Metabolism, 55,* 229–243.

Mink, M., Evans, A., Moore, C. G., Calderon, K. S., & Deger, S. (2010). Nutritional imbalance endorsed by television food advertisements. *Journal of the American Dietetic Association, 110,* 904–910.

Monteiro, P. O., & Victora, C. G. (2005). Rapid growth in infancy and childhood and obesity in later life: A systematic review. *Obesity Reviews, 6,* 143–154.

Moran, C. N., Vassilopoulos, C., Tsiokanos, A., Jamurtas, A. Z., Bailey, M. E., Montgomery, H. E., ... Pitsiladis, Y. P. (2006). The associations of ACE polymorphisms with physical, physiological and skill parameters in adolescents. *European Journal of Human Genetics, 14*(3), 332–339.

Morland, K., Wing, S., Diez Roux, A., & Poole, C. (2002). Neighborhood characteristics associated with the location of food stores and food service places. *American Journal of Preventive Medicine, 22,* 23–29.

Mustelin, L., Silventoinen, K., Pietilainen, K., Rissanen, A., & Kaprio, J. (2008). Physical activity reduces the influence of genetic effects on BMI and waist circumference: A study in young adult twins. *International Journal of Obesity, 33,* 29–36.

Mutch, D. M., & Clement, K. (2006). Genetics of human obesity. *Best Practices in Research and Clinical Endocrinology and Metabolism, 20,* 647–664.

Nader, P. R., O'Brien, M., Houts, R., Bradley, R., Belsky, J., Crosnoe, R., ... Susman, E. J. (2005). Identifying risk for obesity in early childhood. *Pediatrics, 118*(3), e595–e601.

Neel, J. V. (1962). Diabetes mellitus a "thrifty" genotype rendered detrimental by "progress"? *American Journal of Human Genetics, 14,* 352–353.

Nelson, M. C., Gordon-Larsen, P., Song, Y., & Popkin, B. M. (2006). Built and social environments: Associations with adolescent overweight and activity. *American Journal of Preventive Medicine, 31*(2), 109–117.

Newell, A., Zlot, A., Silvey, K., & Ariail, K. (2007). Addressing the obesity epidemic: Genomics perspective. *Preventing Chronic Disease, 4*(2), 1–6.

Newnham, J. P., Pennell, C. E., Lye, S. J., Rampono, J., & Challis, J. R. G. (2009). Early life origins of obesity. *Obstetrics and Gynecology Clinics of North America, 36*, 227–244.

Nicklas, T. A., Baranowski, T., Cullen, K. W., & Berenson, G. (2001). Eating patterns, dietary quality and obesity. *Journal of the American College of Nutrition, 20*(6), 599–608.

Nielsen, S. J., & Popkin, B. M. (2003). Patterns and trends in food portion sizes, 1977–1998. *Journal of the American Medical Association, 289*(4), 450–453.

Nielsen, S. J., & Popkin, B. M. (2004). Changes in beverage intake between 1977 and 2001. *American Journal of Preventive Medicine, 27*, 205–210.

Oken, E., Levitan, E. B., & Gillman, M. W. (2008). Maternal smoking during pregnancy and child overweight: Systematic review and meta-analysis. *International Journal of Obesity, 32*(2), 201–210.

Oken, E., Taveras, E. M., Kleinman, K. P., Rich-Edwards, J. W., & Gillman, M. W. (2007). Gestational weight gain and child adiposity at age 3 years. *American Journal of Obstetrics and Gynecology, 196*, 322e1–322e8.

Ong, K., & Loos, R. (2006). Rapid infancy weight gain and subsequent obesity: Systematic reviews and hopeful suggestions. *Acta Paediatrica, 95*, 904–908.

O'Rahilly, S., & Farooqi, I. S. (2006). Genetics of obesity. *Philosophical Transactions of the Royal Society of London, 361*, 1095–1105.

O'Rahilly, S., Farooqi, I. S., Yeo, G. S., & Challis, B. G. (2003). Minireview: Human obesity: Lessons from monogenic disorders. *Endocrinology, 144*(9), 3757–3764.

Owen, C. G., Martin, R. M., Whincup, P. H., Davey-Smith, G., Gillman, M. W., & Cook, D. G. (2005). The effect of breastfeeding on mean body mass index throughout life: A quantitative review of published and unpublished observational evidence. *American Journal of Clinical Nutrition, 82*, 1298–1307.

Paracchini, V., Pedotti, P., & Taioli, E. (2005). Genetics of leptin and obesity: A HuGE review. *American Journal of Epidemiology, 162*(2), 101–114.

Paeratakul, S., Ferdinand, D. P., Champagne, C. M., Ryan, D. H., & Bray, G. A. (2003). Fast-food consumption among US adults and children: Dietary and nutrient intake profile. *Journal of the American Dietetic Association, 103*(10), 1332–1338.

Patrick, H., & Nicklas, T. A. (2005). A review of family and social determinants of children's eating patterns and diet quality. *Journal of the American College of Nutrition, 24*(2), 83–92.

Piernas, C., & Popkin, B. M. (2010a). Snacking increased among U.S. adults between 1977 and 2006. *Journal of Nutrition, 140*(2), 325–332.

Piernas, C., & Popkin, B. M. (2010b). Trends in snacking among U.S. children. *Health Affairs, 29*(3), 398–404.

Plachta-Danielzik, S., Landsberg, B., Bosy-Westphal, A., Johannsen, M., Lange, D., & Muller, M. J. (2008). Energy gain and energy gap in normal-weight children: Longitudinal data of the KOPS. *Obesity, 16*, 777–783.

Pomp, D., & Mohlke, K. L. (2008). Obesity genes: So close and yet so far. *Journal of Biology, 27*, 36.

Popkin, B. M., & Udry, J. R. (1998). Adolescent obesity increases significantly in second and third generation U.S. immigrants: The National Longitudinal Study of Adolescent Health. *The Journal of Nutrition, 128*(4), 701–706.

Powell, L. M., Chaloupka, F. J., & Bao, Y. (2007). The availability of fast-food and full-service restaurants in the United States: Associations with neighborhood characteristics. *American Journal of Preventive Medicine, 33*(4 Suppl.), S240–S245.

Powell, L. M., Szczypka, G., & Chaloupka, F. J. (2007). Exposure to food advertising on television among US children. *Archives of Pediatric and Adolescent Medicine, 161*(6), 553–560.

Powell, L. M., Szczypka, G., Chaloupka, F. J., & Braunschweig, C. L. (2007). Nutritional content of television food advertisments seen by children and adolescents in the United States. *Pediatrics, 120*(3), 576–583.

Prentice, A. M. (2005). Early influences on human energy regulation: Thrifty genotypes and thrifty phenotypes. *Physiology & Behavior, 86*, 640–645.

Prentice, A. M. (2006). The emerging epidemic of obesity in developing countries. *International Journal of Epidemiology, 35*, 93–99.

Rankinen, T., Zuberi, A., Chagnon, Y. C., Weisnagel, S. J., Argyropoulos, G., Walts, B., . . . Bouchard, C. (2006). The human obesity gene map: The 2005 update. *Obesity (Silver Spring, Md.), 14*(4), 529–644.

Ravussin, E., & Bogardus, C. (2000). Energy balance and weight regulation: Genetics versus environment. *British Journal of Nutrition, 83* (Suppl. 1), S17–S20.

Ravussin, E., Valencia, M. E., Esparza, J., Bennett, P. H., & Schulz, L. O. (1994). Effects of a traditional lifestyle on obesity in Pima Indians. *Diabetes Care, 17*(9), 1067–1074.

Reilly, J. J., Armstrong, J., Dorosty, A. R., Emmett, P. M., Ness, A., Rogers, I.,...Sherriff, A. (2005). Early life risk factors for obesity in childhood: Cohort study. *British Medical Journal (Clinical Research Ed.), 330*(7504), 1357.

Robinson, T. N., Borzekowski, D. L., Matheson, D. M., & Kraemer, H. C. (2007). Effects of fast food branding on young children's taste preferences. *Archives of Pediatric and Adolescent Medicine, 161,* 792–797.

Romao, I., & Roth, J. (2008). Genetic and environmental interactions in obesity and type 2 diabetes. *Journal of the American Dietetic Association, 108,* S24–S28.

Romeis, J. C., Grant, J. D., Knopik, V. S., Pedersen, N. L., & Heath, A. C. (2004). The genetics of middle-age spread in middle-class males. *Twin Research, 7,* 596–602.

Rosenheck, R. (2008). Fast food consumption and increased caloric intake: A systematic review of a trajectory toward weight gain and obesity risk. *Obesity Reviews, 9,* 535–547.

Rozin, P., Dow, S., Moscovitch, M., & Rajaram, S. (1998). What causes humans to begin and end a meal? A role for memory for what has been eaten, as evidenced by a study of multiple meal eating in amnesic patients. *Psychological Science, 9,* 392–396.

Sallis, J. F., & Glanz, K. (2006). The role of built environments in physical activity, eating and obesity in childhood. *The Future of Children, 16,* 89–108.

Sanghavi-Goel, M., McCarthy, E. P., Phillips, R. S., & Wee, C. C. (2004). Obesity among U.S. immigrant subgroups by duration of residence. *Journal of the American Medical Association, 292*(23), 2860–2867.

Santini, F., Maffei, M., Pelosini, C., Salvetti, G., Scartabelli, G., & Pinchera, A. (2009). Melanocortin-4 receptor mutations in obesity. *Advances in Clinical Chemistry, 48,* 95–109.

Schoeller, D. A., & Buchholz, A. C. (2005). Energetics of obesity and weight control: Does diet composition matter? *Journal of the American Dietetic Association, 105,* S24–S28.

Schonemann, P. H. (1997). On models and muddles of heritability. *Genetica, 99,* 97–108.

Schousboe, K., Willemsen, G., Kyvik, K. O., Mortensen, J., Boomsma, D. I., Cornes, B. K., ... Harris, J. R. (2003). Sex differences in heritability of BMI: A comparative study of results from twin studies in eight countries. *Twin Research*, 6(5), 409–421.

Schmitz, K. H., Jacobs, D. R., Schreiner, P. J., & Sternfeld, B. (2000). Physical activity and body weight: Association over ten years in the CARDIA study. *International Journal of Obesity*, 24, 1475–1487.

Schulz, L. O., Bennett, P. H., Ravussin, E., Kidd, J. R., Kidd, K. K., Esparza, J., & Valencia, M. E. (2006). Effects of traditional and western environments on prevalence of type 2 diabetes in Pima Indians in Mexico and the U.S. *Diabetes Care*, 29(8), 1866–1871.

Sealy, Y. (2010). Parents' perceptions of food availability: Implications for childhood obesity. *Social Work in Health Care*, 49(6), 565–580.

Shiv, B., & Fedorikhin, A. (1999). Heart and mind in conflict: The interplay of affect and cognition in consumer decision making. *Journal of Consumer Research*, 26, 278–292.

Silventoinen, K., Rokholm, B., Kaprio, J., & Sorensen, T. I. A. (2010). The genetic and environmental influences on childhood obesity: A systematic review of twin and adoption studies. *International Journal of Obesity*, 34, 29–40.

Simonen, R. L., Rankinen, T., Perusse, L., Rice, T., Rao, D. C., Chagnon, Y., & Bouchard, C. (2003). Genome-wide linkage scan for physical activity levels in the Quebec Family study. *Medicine and Science in Sports and Exercise*, 35(8), 1355–1359.

Snyder, E. E., Walts, B., Pérusse, L., Chagnon, Y. C., Weisnagel, S. J., Rankinen, T., & Bouchard, C. (2004). The human obesity gene map: The 2003 update. *Obesity Research*, 12(3), 369–439.

Sobal, J., & Wansink, B. (2007). Kitchenscapes, tablescapes, platescapes, and foodscapes. *Environment and Behavior*, 39, 124–142.

Sorensen, L. B., Moller, P., Flint, A., Martens, M., & Raben, A. (2003). Effect of sensory perception of foods on appetite and food intake: A review of studies on humans. *International Journal of Obesity*, 27, 1152–1166.

Spalding, K. L., Arner, E., Westermark, P. O., Bernard, S., Buchholz, B. A., Bergmann, O., ... Arner, P. (2008). Dynamics of fat cell turnover in humans. *Nature*, 453(7196), 783–787.

Speakman, J. R. (2004). Obesity: The integrated roles of environment and genetics. *Journal of Nutrition*, 134, 2090S–2105S.

Sternfeld, B., Wang, H., Quesenberry, C. P., Abrams, B., Everson-Rose, S. A., Greendale, G. A., ... Sowers, M. (2004). Physical activity and changes in weight and waist circumference in midlife women: Findings from the Study of Women's Health Across the Nation. *American Journal of Epidemiology, 160*(9), 912–922.

Stettler, N. (2007). Nature and strength of epidemiological evidence for origins of childhood and adulthood obesity in the first year of life. *International Journal of Obesity, 31,* 1035–1043.

Stewart, H., Blisard, N., & Jolliffe, D. (2006). *Let's eat out: Americans weigh taste, convenience, and nutrition.* Washington, DC: US Department of Agriculture Economic Research Service. Retrieved March 7, 2010, from http://www.ers.usda.gov/publications/eib19/eib19.pdf

Stone, S., Abkevich, V., Russell, D. L., Riley, R., Timms, K., Tran, T., ... Shattuck, D. (2006). TBC1D1 is a candidate for a severe obesity gene and evidence for a gene/gene interaction in obesity predisposition. *Human Molecular Genetics, 15*(18), 2709–2720.

St. Onge, M. P., Keller, K. L., & Heymsfield, S. B. (2003). Changes in childhood food consumption patterns: A cause for concern in light of increasing body weights. *American Journal of Clinical Nutrition, 78*(6), 1068–1073.

St. Onge, M. P., Rubiano, F., DeNino, W. F., Jones, A., Greenfield, D., Ferguson, P. W., ... Heymsfield, S. B. (2004). Added thermogenic and satiety effects of a mixed nutrient vs a sugar-only beverage. *International Journal of Obesity and Related Metabolic Disorders, 28*(2), 248–253.

Story, M., Kaphingst, K. M., Robinson-O'Brien, R., & Glanz, K. (2008). Creating healthy food and eating environments: Policy and environmental approaches. *Annual Reviews of Public Health, 29,* 253–72.

Stroebele, N., & De Castro, J. M. (2004). Effect of ambience on food intake and food choice. *Nutrition, 20,* 821–838.

Stunkard, A. J., Foch, T. T., & Hrubec, Z. (1986). A twin study of human obesity. *Journal of the American Medical Association, 256*(1), 51–54.

Stunkard, A. J., Harris, J. R., Pedersen, N. L., & McClearn, G. E. (1990). The body-mass index of twins who have been reared apart. *New England Journal of Medicine, 322*(21), 1483–1487.

Stunkard, A. J., Sørensen, T. I., Hanis, C., Teasdale, T. W., Chakraborty, R., Schull, W. J., & Schulsinger, F. (1986). An adoption study of human obesity. *The New England Journal of Medicine, 314*(4), 193–198.

Tankó, L. B., Siddiq, A., Lecoeur, C., Larsen, P. J., Christiansen, C., Walley, A., & Froguel, P. (2005). ACDC/adiponectin and PPAR-gamma gene polymorphisms: Implications for features of obesity. *Obesity Research, 13*(12), 2113–2121.

Taveras, E. M., Gillman, M. W., Kleinman, K., Rich-Edwards, J. W., & Rifas-Shiman, S. L. (2010). Racial/ethnic differences in early-life risk factors for childhood obesity. *Pediatrics, 125*(4), 1–10.

Taveras, E. M., Rifas-Shiman, S. L., Oken, E., Gunderson, E. P., & Gillman, M. W. (2008). Short sleep duration in infancy and risk of childhood overweight. *Archives of Pediatric and Adolescent Medicine, 162*(4), 305–311.

Taveras, E. M., Rifas-Shiman, S. L., Scanlon, K. S., Grummer-Strawn, L. M., Sherry, B., & Gillman, M. W. (2006). To what extent is the protective effect of breastfeeding on future overweight explained by decreased maternal feeding restriction? *Pediatrics, 118*(6), 2341–2348.

Tudor-Locke, C., Kronenfeld, J. J., Kim, S. S., Benin, M., & Kuby, M. (2007). A geographical comparison of prevalence of overweight school-aged children: The National Survey of Children's Health 2003. *Pediatrics, 120*(4), 1043–1050.

U.S. Department of Agriculture, Agricultural Research Service, Beltsville Human Nutrition Research Center, Food Surveys Research Group. (2010). Snacking patterns of U.S. adolescents: What we eat in America, NHANES 2005–2006. *Food Surveys Research Group Dietary Data Brief.* Retrieved December 13, 2010, from http://ars.usda.gov/Services/docs.htm?docid=19476

van Erk, M. J., Blom, W. A., vanOmmen, B., & Hendriks, H. F. (2006). High-protein and high-carbohydrate breakfasts differentially change the transcriptome of human blood cells. *American Journal of Clinical Nutrition, 84,* 1233–1241.

van Harmelen, V., Skurk, T., Röhrig, K., Lee, Y. M., Halbleib, M., Aprath-Husmann, I., & Hauner, H. (2003). Effect of BMI and age on adipose tissue cellularity and differentiation capacity in women. *International Journal of Obesity and Related Metabolic Disorders, 27*(8), 889–895.

Vartanian, L. R., Herman, C. P., & Polivy, J. (2007). Consumption stereotypes and impression management: How you are what you eat. *Appetite, 48,* 265–277.

Walley, A. J., Asher, J. E., & Froguel, P. (2009). The genetic contribution to non-syndromic human obesity. *Nature Reviews/Genetics*, *10*, 431–442.

Wang, Y. C., Gortmaker, S. L., Sobol, A. M., & Kuntz, K. M. (2006). Estimating the energy gap among US children: A counterfactual approach. *Pediatrics*, *118*(6), e1721–1733.

Wansink, B. (2004). Environmental factors that increase the food intake and consumption volume of unknowing consumers. *Annual Reviews in Nutrition*, *24*, 455–479.

Wansink, B., & Cheney, M. M. (2005). Super bowls: Serving bowl size and food consumption. *Journal of the American Medical Association*, *293*, 1727–1728.

Wansink, B., & Kim, J. (2004). Bad popcorn in big buckets: Portion size can influence intake as much as taste. *Journal of Nutrition Education and Behavior*, *37*(5), 242–245.

Wansink, B., Painter, J. E., & Lee, Y. K. (2006). The office candy dish: Proximity's influence on estimated and actual consumption. *International Journal of Obesity*, *30*, 871–875.

Wansink, B., & Wansink, C. S. (2010). The largest Last Supper: Depictions of food portions and plate size increased over the millennium. *International Journal of Obesity*, *34*, 943–944.

Wardle, J., & Carnell, S. (2009). Appetite is a heritable phenotype associated with adiposity. *Annals of Behavioral Medicine*, *38*(Suppl. 1), S25–S30.

Wardle, J., Carnell, S., Haworth, C., & Plomin, R. (2008). Evidence for a strong genetic influence on childhood adiposity despite the force of the obesogenic environment. *American Journal of Clinical Nutrition*, *87*, 398–404.

Wardle, J., Herrera, M. L., Cooke, L., & Gibson, E. L. (2003). Modifying children's food preferences: The effects of exposure and reward on acceptance of an unfamiliar vegetable. *European Journal of Clinical Nutrition*, *57*(2), 341–348.

Welsh, J. A., Cogswell, M. E., Rogers, S., Rockett, H., Mei, Z., & Grummer-Strawn, L. M. (2005). Overweight among low-income preschool children associated with the consumption of sweet drinks: Missouri, 1999–2002. *Pediatrics*, *115*(2), e223–e229.

Westerterp-Plantenga, M. S. (2004). Effects of energy density of daily food intake on long-term energy intake. *Physiology & Behavior*, *81*, 765–771.

Whitaker, R. C. (2004). Predicting preschooler obesity at birth: The role of maternal obesity in early pregnancy. *Pediatrics, 114*, e29–e36.

Woodward-Lopez, G., Kao, J., & Ritchi, L. (2010). To what extent have sweetened beverages contributed to the obesity epidemic? *Public Health Nutrition*, 1–11.

World Health Organization. (2000). *Obesity: Preventing and managing the global epidemic* (WHO Technical Report Series, 894). Geneva, Switzerland: Author.

Young, L. R., & Nestle, M. (2007). Portion sizes and obesity: Responses of fast-food companies. *Journal of Public Health Policy, 28*, 238–248.

3

Psychosocial Correlates and Consequences of Obesity

educing the psychological and social impacts of obesity into a single chapter is a challenge. This is largely due to the complex interactions among obesity and one's personality, environment, preexisting conditions or psychopathology, age, gender, race or ethnicity, geographic location, and lifestyle, to name a few. Perhaps the greatest challenge is determining whether a psychosocial concern is a result of obesity, a cause of obesity, or simply a factor that correlates by virtue of some external variable. For example, as you read on, you will see how difficult it is to tease out whether people become depressed as a result of their obesity and low self-image; if people experiencing depression tend to overeat and have limited activity, leading to weight gain; or if some other factor leads to both depression and obesity, such as an underactive thyroid or a history of childhood maltreatment. Therefore, while it's important to look at correlations with obesity, it's also important that we try our best to interpret them correctly, which means not assuming that one thing causes another just because they co-occur. So, before we start discussing the history of the psychological and social impacts of obesity, we'd like to briefly discuss why *correlation does not imply causation*.

If you've had to sit through this discussion in an introductory statistics class at some point, then feel free to skip this paragraph—our feelings will only be slightly hurt. When two variables are correlated, it may be easy to jump to the conclusion that one of those factors caused the other. For example, there is a correlation between ice cream sales and the average amount of people going to the beach. Could you say that the act of purchasing ice cream actually causes people to go to the beach? Conversely, could you say that going to the beach causes people to buy ice cream? Obviously, the answer is no, or at least, not directly. It is more likely that some outside variable, such as high temperatures and time off from work or school (i.e., summertime), has caused these outcomes. Still, they are often associated in some way, and that can still give us some important information. Good—now we can move on.

A HISTORY OF THE PSYCHOSOCIAL IMPACTS OF OBESITY

It's likely that the medical consequences of obesity have not changed dramatically over time. In fact, as early as 600 BC, an Indian physician known as Sushruta wrote of the medical correlates of obesity, such as chest pain and heart problems (Dwivedi & Dwivedi, 2007). However, the negative psychological and social consequences have varied somewhat. For one, obese sculptures and drawings dating back from 8000 to 5500 BC are believed to have been created as a representation of a bountiful harvest and fertility (Wolin & Petrelli, 2009). One need only look in an art museum to see depictions of obese women, such as the works of Rubens, representing an ideal image of female beauty hundreds of years ago. In addition, it is well known that obesity was previously viewed as a sign of wealth and status during the Middle Ages, and even still today in some parts of Africa, the Polynesian islands, or areas where food is scarce. This is likely due to differences in the availability of food, which is a problem that has essentially disappeared in modern industrialized societies. Where food is scarce, it would be a sign of prestige to maintain a higher weight, as it signaled the individual could afford plenty of food. It was also a sign that those individuals did not need to perform manual labor; in other words, they did not need to be active and exert energy to either procure their own food or earn a living.

Still, many ancient cultures viewed obesity as a problem, including Ancient Egyptians and Ancient Tibetans (Wolin & Petrelli, 2009). Buddhists in the 12th century viewed obesity as the result of moral failure (Stunkard, LaFleur, & Wadden, 1998). The negative societal views of obesity also can be linked to religious fervor. In early Christian times, the first version of the Cardinal Sins, or Seven Deadly Sins, provided a guide for the most objectionable of acts, and gluttony made the cut. The overconsumption or excessive indulgence in food was viewed by Catholics, who represented much of society, as a pretty serious weakness of character. Throughout history, perceptions of obesity have varied, and with those changes in perception we have seen changes in the psychological and social consequences of obesity.

Flash forward a bit to the 1920s. Our grandmother (technically Eric's, although she has taken on the role with Lauren as well), now at age 86, remains one of the most intelligent people we know. This has been evident through conversation, her ability to quickly complete any Sudoku or crossword puzzle, and her performance on individually administered cognitive ability and achievement tests, which she happily volunteered for in exchange for a visit from her grandchild in graduate school many years ago. Nonetheless, as a young girl in the 1920s, her mother's friends used to believe that she was "retarded" (as our grandmother tells it) for no other reason than the fact that she was overweight. In her retelling of the story, her mother brought her to the doctor at the constant urging of her mother's friends to inquire about our grandmother's mental state. The doctor asked her some questions and then stepped out of the office briefly. He returned with a colleague who was described by our grandmother as a "short, round man," at which point the doctor said something to the effect of, "This man is one of the most accomplished physicians in this office. Does he look retarded to you?" We hope this short, round physician had a sense of humor; regardless, he helped prove a point. The doctor then said, "She's not retarded; just stop feeding her."

Our grandmother explains that people didn't routinely exercise just for the sake of exercising when she was a child or young adult, and a typical breakfast consisted of eggs, bacon, sausage, pancakes with syrup, and toast with a nice square of butter on top. The health-conscious individual who wakes up at 5:30 am for a workout, followed by a fruit smoothie with skim milk or a protein bar and a bike ride to work, was uncommon. Until relatively recently, the consequences of our nutritional decisions and activity levels were not as well known or publicized. The conceptualization of a new eating disorder called orthorexia nervosa, which describes an obsession with avoiding unhealthy foods (this is currently not recognized by the *Diagnostic and Statistical Manual*–Fourth Edition [*DSM-IV*]; American Psychiatric Association, 2000), would have been unheard of. Nevertheless, our grandmother's story makes it clear that although most people fell within a relatively "normal" weight, a few were overweight or obese, and they were viewed negatively. As for our grandmother, they thought she was unintelligent simply because she was heavy. Sadly, such misperceptions continue to be a reality.

PERCEPTIONS OF IDEAL WEIGHT

Some attention should be given to changes in *perceptions* of obesity, rather than simply changes in actual rates of objective measures of obesity, in part due to the role that social perception plays in actual psychological and social responses to obesity. Whereas many medical and physical consequences of obesity are more directly related to the physiological dangers of excess body weight, many social and psychological consequences of obesity are related to the perceptions of others. A third-grade classroom exercise referred to as the "brown-eyed/blue-eyed exercise" completed by Jane Elliott in 1968 illustrates this point beautifully.

Jane Elliott wanted to teach her third graders a lesson about the impacts of prejudice, and divided her classroom into two groups—those in the blue-eyed group, and those in the brown-eyed group. She began throwing insults to the children in the brown-eyed group, encouraging the blue-eyed children to join in the fun. Further, she favored the blue-eyed children, giving them extra snacks, more time on the playground, and compliments for effort and intelligence. The two groups could not drink from the same water fountain. She pretended to cite scientific facts that brown-eyed children were inferior in nearly every way imaginable, and made them wear ribbons to further draw out their differences. Amazingly, within the day, the children all followed suit. Those in the blue-eyed group began performing higher academically, and conversely, the brown-eyed group regressed. Further, brown-eyed children sulked, berated themselves, and noted disinterest in coming back to school the next day, whereas the blue-eyed children demonstrated mature, engaged, enthusiastic, positive attitudes towards school. The next day, Jane Elliott reversed the roles after stating she had made a mistake, stating that in fact, the brown-eyed children were superior. While similar behaviors occurred with reversed roles, Jane Elliott reported noticing less intense reactions from the children, which was partly attributed to the experience of having been discriminated against the day before. This classroom based study was described in detail through the films *A Class Divided* (Peters, 1971a) and *Eye of the Storm* (Peters, 1971b).

The remarkable outcome of this classroom experiment highlighted the effect of social roles, how people treat each other, and perceptions on a variety of outcomes, including mood, self-image, academic performance, attitudes, and behaviors. You might imagine that the kind of negative perceptions and social interactions that obese and overweight individuals face could (and does) have a similar influence across a variety of psychosocial outcomes.

Adult attitudes and behaviors are also susceptible to social perceptions and social roles. The Stanford prison experiment completed by psychology professor Philip Zimbardo in 1971 illustrates this point well (Can you tell we like old psychology studies?). Undergraduates were randomly assigned to play the roles of inmates or guards in a mock prison. The guards were instructed to make the inmates feel afraid and powerless, and they played their roles well. The guards became violent, crass, sadistic, and authoritarian towards the inmates. Conversely, the inmates began to suffer from severe emotional stress and internalized their roles as powerless, inferior people. Two inmates had to be removed due to experiencing psychological trauma. The experiment was stopped early after six days. Certainly, this example is extreme, and other factors played a role in the participants' behavior, although it illustrates the impact of the perceptions of others on behavior and how people treat one another.

Now that we all agree that perceptions can impact psychosocial consequences, lets discuss how perceptions of beauty and obesity have changed, even within recent history. Many of us have heard the phrase, "beauty is in the eye of the beholder." Well, the beholders of beauty, and their perceptions of ideal body weight, have changed over time, and are dependent on many factors, including culture, racial and ethnic identification, and gender. As for Caucasian women, consider one of the most desired women in the 1950s, Marilyn Monroe. Marilyn Monroe was a size 14—and was approximately 5'5" and weighed between 118 and 135 pounds. She was eventually replaced in the 1960s by models such as Twiggy, who was 5'6" and weighed around 90 pounds, or the infamous Barbie doll. Many often talk about Barbie setting unrealistic standards for beauty, given that if she were full size she would be 5'9", 110 pounds (more than 30 pounds underweight), and would have a nearly impossible bust-to-waist-to-hip ratio of 36-18-33. Brownell and Napolitano (1995) found that for a healthy adult woman to meet Barbie's standards, she would have to grow five inches in the chest, more than 3 inches in neck length, all while dropping 6 inches in the waist. In 1965, a Barbie doll came adorned with a book titled "How to Lose Weight," with a short but helpful tip included— "Don't eat." In the 1990s, the creators of Barbie finally buckled and made her proportions more within the realm of possible, although don't expect to see "Curvy Barbie" in stores anytime soon. Although we cannot place all the blame on Barbie and her impossible standard of beauty, what we are left with currently is the fact that *most* women, including those of normal weight, believe that they would need to lose weight in order to be attractive, and most are currently trying to lose weight (Cook, MacPherson, & Langille, 2007; Malinauskas, Raedeke, Aeby, Smith, & Dallas, 2006). In other words, normal-weight women frequently think they are overweight, which can lead to a high degree of psychosocial problems as well as increased risk of eating disorders. Perhaps, the standards for beauty have become a bit too narrow (no pun intended)?

The picture is not quite so simplistic, however. For example, the perceptions of what makes women attractive to adolescent men differ based on race, with African American males pre-ferring larger body sizes (Adams et al., 2000; Jones, Fries, & Danish, 2007). Also, consider a recent study of inner city, African American children of poor socioeconomic status (SES) that revealed the majority of both the children and the parents in these communities viewed overweight children as being at a normal and healthy weight (Skelton, Busey, & Havens, 2006). For the population in this study, being overweight or even slightly obese was actually perceived as "normal" within their culture or community. Thus, the psychosocial impacts of obe-sity (e.g., low self-esteem, poor body image, risk of disordered eating) were likely reduced. One negative consequence in such cases, is that it's likely that efforts to lose weight and develop a healthier lifestyle are also reduced (He & Evans, 2007).

In contrast, in cities in China, one study found that most boys viewed themselves as too thin (Xie et al., 2006) even if they were at normal weight; and females in this study thought they were overweight even if they weren't. Generally, misperception of weight status appears to occur more frequently among racial/ethnic minorities, males, and individuals with lower education (Dorsey, Eberhardt, & Ogden, 2009). Although we won't get into all of the specifics of different views of ideal body weight within different groups, the point is clear: perceptions are important to the psychosocial impacts of obesity, and those perceptions are not static over time or population.

CURRENT PSYCHOLOGICAL AND SOCIAL CORRELATES OF OBESITY

In the late 20th and early 21st centuries, it seems that Americans have developed somewhat bipolar views toward eating, activity, and weight. On the one hand, we face a constant barrage of efforts to get us to eat and drink more (e.g., TV ads, supersize portions in restaurants). On the other hand, we are constantly being told that we need to lose weight through the latest fad diet in order to look like, and be as successful as, Brad Pitt and Angelina Jolie (fine, so maybe we'll never look like celebrities, but you get the point). One minute, you hear reports about the dangers of obesity, and the next minute you hear organizations such as the National Association to Advance Fat Acceptance (www.naafa.org) fighting to end weight-based discrimination and providing a message that people should accept their bodies the way they are and be happy. Overindulgence in almost anything is often viewed as a weakness in character and can result in ridicule or prejudice. But then we are confronted with scenarios where overindulgence is glorified and even rewarded. For example, hot dog eating contests promote consuming enormous amounts of food at once, and as of the writing of this book, the current champion, Joey Chestnut, recently consumed 68 hot dogs in 10 minutes and won a substantial amount of cash for the effort. Others may watch shows on television that promote other eating contests, where individuals (usually men) are cheered and applauded for consuming tens of thousands of calories in a single serving. For the rest of us, the stigma associated with obesity can be very serious. In fact, "...stigmatization of obese individuals poses serious risks to their psychological and physical health, generates health disparities, and interferes with implementation of effective obesity prevention efforts" (Puhl & Heuer, 2010, p. 1019). Further, following a survey of school-aged children, Rimm (2004) notes, "for every single social-emotional variable related to children's worries and confidence, overweight children fared worse than those of average weight" (p. 34).

While maintaining the notion that correlation does not imply causation, we intend to break down the various consequences that are often associated with obesity, and how gender, racial or ethnic subgroup, age, and other variables may influence those consequences. However, before doing so, we will first discuss theories related to how social groups may promote the transmission of obesity.

SOCIAL TRANSMISSION OF OBESITY

As stated throughout this book, and throughout every textbook, magazine, and journal article related to nutrition or weight, obesity has increased significantly within the past few decades across our entire society. Such a sharp increase cannot be due solely to genetics; thus, we look to aspects of society or our environment to see why this has happened.

Christakis and Fowler (2007) set out to shed light on this issue, hypothesizing that the looks of those we spend time with impact our own weight gain. Comparisons can be drawn to someone who spends a lot of time with friends who drink alcohol, smoke cigarettes, run a lot, play ultimate Frisbee, watch NASCAR, and so on; we tend to adapt our interests to those of our friends and social networks. We like spending time with people who are like us. The authors also postulated that spending time with obese or overweight friends may increase our own tolerance for being obese.

They evaluated a group of 12,067 individuals over a period of 32 years (and yes, they used BMI as a weight indicator), and found that indeed, obesity can be spread through our social networks. Here is what they found more specifically:

- Chances of obesity increased by 57% for those who had obese friends; however,
  - for mutual friends (i.e., that person identifies you as a friend as well), the increase in risk was 171%;
  - when the obese individuals thought they were friends with the individuals in the study, although the study participant didn't view the obese person as a friend, the increased risk was negligible.
- Chances of obesity increased by 40% if an adult sibling became obese.
- Chances of obesity increased by 37% if someone's spouse became obese.

- Closeness of the relationship had more of an impact on social transmission than geographic distance.
  - For example, having an obese neighbor had negligible impact on risk.
  - Individuals of the same sex had more impact on each other than the opposite sex.

Taken a step further, across the entire study, having direct association with an obese individual increased the risk of obesity by 45%. Having two degrees of separation (friend of a friend who is obese) increased the risk by 20%. Three degrees of separation increased the risk by 10%. Risk was negligible at four degrees.

Additional research has supported these claims; for example, children with two obese parents have an increased risk of obesity (Whitaker, Jarvis, Beeken, Boniface, & Wardle, 2010). Risk goes up if both parents are severely obese. (Of course, genetics plays a role here as well.) Taken together, this important research suggests that although obesity is often viewed as causing various psychosocial consequences, the relationship is a two-way street. Our social ties can have consequences for our weight and health. Our health, our behavior, and our weight are unquestionably related to our social networks.

Importantly, some research has actually challenged the claims made by Christakis and Fowler, implying that errors were made in the original analysis (Cohen-Cole & Fletcher, 2008). They claim that community-level and "shared environmental factors can cause the appearance of social network effects" (p. 1386). In other words, you are more likely to be close friends with someone who lives near you and shares the same socioeconomic environment, lives near the same food stores, and maybe even has a similar job to you. It may actually be that these shared environments predispose people to gain weight. So although Cohen-Cole and Fletcher don't deny that social networks impact obesity, they *significantly* downplay the strength of those effects, noting that some of the effects are negligible and not significant.

I know, it's difficult to know what to believe and how to tease out the most important findings. It's OK, you're not alone. Welcome to the wonderful world of the social sciences.

SOCIAL PREJUDICE AND DISCRIMINATION

Before reading any further, I challenge you to honestly consider your own views of obesity. How do you view overweight or obese individuals? What reaction do you have when you see an extremely obese person sitting next to you at the movies? On a plane? At a restaurant? Does this vary based on age, gender, racial or ethnic group, location, wealth, or any other factors? Do you view an individual's obesity and weight as within his or her personal control? Have you ever thought, "They should just stop eating so much, or they should just hit the gym"? What do you think when you see an obese child? Perhaps, you blame the parent, or consider the child weak or impulsive. Maybe, you assume he gets bullied on the playground or has no friends. Whether you care to admit it or not, most people (we're talking probably close to 99.99% here) make these sort of snap judgments. The fact is, most us have these sorts of implicit biases against obese people, often despite our best intentions. Although many would like to think that they see beauty from the inside, research suggests otherwise.

The prevalence of obesity continues to rise, and with it, so does the prevalence of discrimination against obesity. In fact, prejudice against obesity is considered as common as racial prejudice (Puhl, Andreyeva, & Brownell, 2008). Perhaps more alarming is the finding from a study in 1967 (Staffieri) that 6-year-old children described pictures of overweight children using adjectives such as lazy, dirty, stupid, ugly, cheats, and liars. Other studies have suggested that such views are present as early as 3 years of age (Cramer & Steinwert, 1998). It's hard to tell whether such opinions are a product of our society, some universal characteristic among most humans leading us to stigmatize those who are different from us, or a little of both. What remains clear is that social prejudice and discrimination against the overweight and obese begin pretty early.

Additional studies have found similar trends among college students and adults. One study in particular (Vener, Krupka, & Gerard, 1982) found that college students viewed obese individuals as less preferable as marriage partners in relation to cocaine users, shoplifters, and embezzlers. What may be particularly alarming is a study in 2003 (Schwartz, Chambliss, Brownell, Blair, & Billington) that found significant weight bias among health care professionals. What was most striking about this study was that the health care professionals were all involved in obesity treatment! Such biases can lead to serious additional consequences for obese individuals, most notably a reduction in quality care from health care providers.

What's worse is that such perceptions often lead to weight-based stigmatization, which leads to a host of other negative outcomes, including binge eating and unhealthy weight control behaviors (Puhl & Heuer, 2010). Believe it or not, some still believe that applying weight-based stigma may actually motivate obese individuals to exercise and eat healthier—yet research evidence contradicts this notion (e.g., Libbey, Story, Neumark-Sztainer, & Boutelle, 2008; Neumark-Sztainer et al., 2002). As a rule, demoralizing people is not a good motivator.

Weight-based stigmatization is frequent and occurs across various aspects of society. Consider the continuing saga of whether to charge obese individuals extra money to fly on commercial airlines. Now, from an economic standpoint, the move to charge extra makes some sense. It was estimated that the average weight gain during the 1990s actually cost airlines an additional $275 million and 1.3 billion additional liters of fuel (Yee, 2004). So, their solution was to increase fares across the board. Further, airlines began charging the cost of two seats to passengers who can't lower both armrests, in part to provide safe and comfortable seating. This has caused considerable controversy, as some refer to it as discrimination. Nonetheless, many major commercial airlines continue to post on their Web sites that any passenger who can't lower both armrests must buy two seats. Discrimination? Maybe. Stigmatizing and degrading? Certainly.

Another example comes from a large number of studies that have convincingly found that unattractive and overweight defendants in a court of law tend to receive longer sentences and more frequent convictions than more attractive defendants, given the same facts and evidence (e.g., Gunnell & Ceci, 2010). This is interesting given that Lady Justice, the Roman goddess of justice, comes with three symbols of the rule of law, one of which is a blindfold representing objective impartiality. Go figure.

These examples simply suggest that overweight or obese people face a lot of discrimination and prejudice. These biases can lead to negative occupational and educational outcomes.

OCCUPATIONAL DISCRIMINATION

In the job market, obese people are less likely to be hired, promoted, or receive a positive performance rating, with all other things being equal. Obesity appears to lead to lower income as well, although there are some group differences there. Some of these differences were highlighted by Mark Roehling (1999) in a review of almost 30 different studies:

- Occupational discrimination appears to be more of a problem for women than men.
  - Obese Caucasian women earn 5.9% less than normal-weight women
  - Morbidly obese Caucasian women earned 24.1% less

- Men's wages were not as impacted by weight.
  - In fact, mildly obese Caucasian and African American men earned *more* than normal-weight men
  - Only morbidly obese men earned significantly less
- While obese men are not as heavily penalized in wages, they are under represented in managerial and professional jobs, and over represented in transportation jobs (Puhl & Brownell, 2001).
- Wage differences tend to be more pronounced among Caucasian women; such differences are not as obvious among African American women.

You might be wondering why obesity leads to such lower occupational success, and that would be a good question. Remember, we are not able to conclusively state a cause just because obesity and occupational success are negatively correlated. Perhaps, some individuals with obesity included in these studies legitimately did not perform as well as others, or they did not have the confidence to ask for a raise or even apply for more high-paying jobs. Of course, it could be because employers, in one way or another, applied some social prejudice to their decision making, and several researchers have made that claim. Roehling (1999) noted that obese individuals were often viewed as possessing some negative qualities or personality traits, or were seen as emotionally impaired in some way. There are other factors at play as well, including expected increases in insurance premiums, more frequent absences, and additional costs for accommodations, to name a few.

WHAT'S LAW GOT TO DO WITH IT (GOT TO DO WITH IT)?

Historically, obesity has not technically been covered under disability law unless it's primarily due (with evidence) to some psychological or physiological condition (such as an underactive thyroid, for example). As you may or may not know, written law is eventually interpreted by case law in the courts, where individual rulings set precedents for future lawsuits. Although there is an extensive history of case law related to obesity discrimination, we provide merely a summary of some of the important changes that have impacted and will continue to impact obesity discrimination in the workplace.[1]

- Title VII of the Civil Rights Act prohibits discrimination based on race, color, religion, sex, and nationality but not weight specifically.
- The Americans with Disabilities Act of 1990 (ADA) requires employers to not discriminate against, and provide appropriate accommodations for, individuals with disabilities. ADA defines a disability as a physical or mental impairment that substantially limits one or more major life activities. Major life activities include a wide array of tasks, such as sitting, standing, lifting, breathing, walking, seeing, hearing, learning, working, and so on.
- Being overweight is generally not considered a disability under ADA unless the individual can document that it is due to a physiological impairment. The law also specifically states that "normal deviations in weight" are not considered impairments. Therefore, an employment decision or practice based on weight may not be illegal in and of itself.
- Being extremely obese (or having a BMI of at least 40) under ADA is considered an impairment, often because there is an underlying or resulting condition, such as diabetes, heart disease, hypertension, depression, or degenerative arthritis.
- Several court cases interpreted the law such that obesity was often *not* considered a disability, even in the case of extreme obesity.
  - For example, the Equal Employment Opportunity Commission sued Watkins Motor Lines, Inc., in 2005 over their firing of an employee who weighed more than

400 pounds. To make a long story short, Watkins Motor Lines, Inc., hired a man in 1990 who weighed 340 pounds to work as a driver and on a loading dock that required climbing, kneeling, bending, stooping, balancing, reaching, and heavy lifting. His weight ranged up to 450 pounds during his employment. In 1995, the employee was climbing a ladder and the rung broke under his weight, and he hurt his knee. He took a leave of absence, at which point the employer informed him of the company policy that after 180 days of absence, employees are terminated if they can't return to work. Further, in order to come back to work, he would need a release from a doctor. The examining doctor said that although he could do the driving, he could not meet the other requirements of the job. So, Watkins Motor Lines fired him. He sued, saying he was discharged because of his weight, and lost. The court said that obesity, without a physiological cause, is not considered an impairment under ADA. This is despite the fact that the man was in the extreme obesity range based on his BMI (unless he was more than 7 feet tall, which was not mentioned in the court documents).

- There is a stipulation in the law that provides protection if you are "regarded" as having an impairment. In other words, if your employer perceives you as disabled and treats you as such, you can receive protections under ADA. Some cases have gone to court with this claim, although as a whole, very few cases have been successful for the plaintiffs. This is probably because employers can make a case that weight prohibits an individual's ability to carry out certain tasks of a job, such as the case described above.

- Michigan and Massachusetts have enacted laws against weight discrimination, and some municipalities have followed suit, including San Francisco, Santa Cruz, and Washington, DC.

- In September, 2008, the ADA Amendments Act of 2008 (ADAAA) was enacted (effective as of January, 2009), which expands protections available to individuals with disabilities as well as what may constitute a disability, particularly given an expansion of "major life activities." It is more likely that obesity will be covered under ADAAA, although without any recent case law to interpret the written law, it's hard to say definitively as of the writing of this book. Perhaps we can give an answer in the next edition (wink). In the meantime, Thompson (2010, p. 266) states, "an individual with an impairment, including morbid obesity, and possibly simple obesity or obesity-related health conditions that limit a major life activity related to bodily functions, may successfully maintain a claim under ADAAA."

● Traditionally, courts apply the same standards in defining a disability between ADA and Section 504 of the Rehabilitation Act of 1973. Section 504 has significant implications for public schools given that students with a disability may be eligible for accommodations or modifications under this law. Changes made with ADAAA related to obesity may therefore change what supports schools may offer to obese students. Some school districts (e.g., Flagler County, FL; Sevier County, TN) already have policies in place to provide Section 504 accommodations or modifications to obese students.

EDUCATIONAL CORRELATES OF OBESITY

In general, obesity is frequently associated with lower rates of academic success. Recently, a group of researchers (Bethell, Simpson, Stumbo, Carle, & Gombojav, 2010) evaluated data from the 2007 National Survey of Children's Health and found that overweight or obese children were 32% more likely to repeat a grade than their normal-weight peers. Their attendance rates were lower as well. Additional research suggests that overweight children are underrepresented in gifted and talented programs, are less likely to describe themselves as hard workers, are more likely to report that their teachers do not understand them, and are more likely to be enrolled in special education programs due to attention deficit/hyperactivity disorder (ADHD), learning disabilities, or behavioral or emotional disabilities (Rimm, 2004). If you recall the blue-eyed/brown-eyed study example, it makes sense that obese kids may underperform in the face of stigmatization from peers and teachers.

The causal relationships, though, become a little cloudy. For example, overweight and obese children are more likely to be teased or bullied than their normal-weight peers. A recent study found that, despite having good social or academic skills, obese children were 65% more likely to be bullied than normal-weight children (Lumeng et al., 2010). In fact, many remember the tragic story of Megan Meier, a 13-year-old girl who had been cyber-bullied and teased on the Internet, in part for her weight, who eventually hanged herself. We also know that bullying (which includes weight-based teasing) has been linked to numerous negative outcomes, including anxiety, depression, truancy and school dropout, decreased academic performance, negative attitudes about school, less physical activity, less participation in sports, and negative attitudes about sports. So, it's hard to say whether grade retention and lower attendance have to do directly with obesity, or whether it's due to weight-based stigmatization. In fact, it's fair to assume that the relationship between obesity and educational outcomes is largely indirect. What we do know, however, is that school-aged overweight and obese children are significantly more likely to experience difficulties in school, both socially and academically. Even with the knowledge that the relationship may be indirect, these facts are very concerning.

Interestingly, some research has found that overweight and obesity are associated with brain atrophy and smaller brain volume, with reductions in volume of 4% and 8%, respectively (Raji et al., 2009; Ward, Carlsson, Trivedi, Sager, & Johnson, 2005). Now, for those who still believe that we only use 10% of our brains, this may be alarming; luckily that's not true.

However, these findings are still very significant. What's worse is that it affects some critical parts of the brain, including the frontal lobes, anterior cingulate gyrus, hippocampus, basal ganglia, and parietal lobes. If you've glazed over, our brain labeling has stopped (for now), but these areas are responsible for things such as judgment, planning, higher-order reasoning, inhibiting impulses, attention, decision making, memory, processing speed, and sensory integration; all critical skills in learning and overall functioning. We are going to go out on a limb and say that weaknesses in these areas could lead to decreased academic performance.[2]

Additionally, obese school-aged children often face discrimination and bias from educators, administrators, and peers. To start, many believe (us included) that teacher expectations impact actual behavior and performance. If a teacher expects a certain student to fail, then that student is likely to perform poorly. These expectations are often based on appearance. In studies examining educator attitudes towards overweight and obese students, many reported that these students are untidy, less likely to succeed, more emotional, lack self-control, and have underlying psychological problems (Neumark-Sztainer, Story, & Harris, 1999; Puhl & Brownell, 2003). These kinds of negative expectations can have serious effects on student performance.

The relationship between obesity and educational performance gets even more complicated. A great deal of research has linked physical activity to educational performance; exercise has been shown to improve cognitive function, attention, and problem-solving skills (so put a bookmark in and bring this book with you to the treadmill). Exercise also has been found to limit the symptoms of depression, anxiety, ADHD, and stress, while improving learning ability and executive functioning (e.g., planning, initiating tasks, problem solving, shifting attention, inhibiting impulses, etc.). Depression, anxiety, ADHD, and stress can often negatively influence educational functioning. So, if obesity leads to decreased physical activity, then maybe that contributes to lower educational outcomes for overweight or obese individuals. Or maybe, just maybe, all these factors are bidirectional, inter-related, and intersect with a host of other variables. Again, the important take-away message is that obesity is often associated with a wide array of negative outcomes, and educational performance is one of them.

When it comes to college attendance, some research has indicated that obese women are only half as likely to attend college when compared with normal-weight women (Crosnoe, 2007), a difference that was more evident in communities where obesity was less prevalent, meaning that obese individuals stood out more. In contrast, college enrollment among men did not differ at all between obese and nonobese populations. This finding led Crosnoe to suggest that women are more vulnerable to decreased self-image and self-concept, and social norms affect educational outcomes for women more so than men. This is not surprising, given the added social pressure on women to be thin.

DEPRESSION

It is often believed that overweight and obese people tend to experience more depression than others. On the surface, this seems to make sense, particularly given the information presented thus far in this chapter. The fact that obesity is often associated with worse outcomes educationally, occupationally, and socially might lead one to believe that depression is an expected, and even likely, outcome of obesity. The conclusion that obesity leads to depression, however, is not necessarily the case; at least, it's not the rule. Truth be told, the relationship between obesity and depression is quite complex. At this point, this shouldn't surprise you.

First, let's briefly discuss depression. Many of us go through moments, minutes, hours, or sometimes even a couple days of a blue or sullen mood. Teenagers may often claim that their world is ending because their boyfriend or girlfriend of nine days was seen kissing someone else in the hallways. You might feel depressed when waking up to an alarm on a Monday morning when it's raining outside. In fact, our dog even seems to get a little down if, for example, we take away her rawhide before she's had enough time to devour it. Fluctuations in mood are normal and do not indicate a disorder. Actual depression, however, is more significant, chronic, encompassing, and pervasive. It can affect every aspect of an individual's life, to the point where he or she has difficulty functioning. In the end, most psychological disorders have this caveat; brief symptoms alone do not dictate a disorder, but if those symptoms are severe enough to cause significant impairments in functioning, then a diagnosis may be warranted.

Specifically, the American Psychiatric Association (APA [*DSM-IV-TR*], 2000) defines major depression as a depressed or irritable mood or loss of interest in previously enjoyable activities for at least a period of two weeks. These symptoms are also accompanied by significant weight loss or weight gain, changes in appetite, changes in sleep patterns, lack of energy, low self-worth poor concentration or decision making, or thoughts of death or suicide. Depression is generally more common among women, although the specific gender differences related to obesity and depression are addressed in more detail below.

Males

So how are obesity and depression related for males? Well, for starters, obese men do not experience depression at a higher rate than nonobese men (except for extremely obese men). In fact, obese men are significantly *less* likely to report a history of depression than average or overweight men. In contrast, underweight men had higher rates of depression and suicidal ideation when compared with average weight men (Carpenter, Hasin,

Allison, & Faith, 2000). SES does not appear to play a role in this relationship either. Importantly, though, extreme obesity in men does correlate significantly with depression. If you think about the social consequences of being obese for males, they seem to parallel this trend with depression, where the impact of being overweight or obese is fairly minimal until you get to the extremely obese category.

Females

Obese female adults have a significantly higher likelihood of depression than normal-weight females, although the degree of significance is not so clear. Female vulnerability to depression and low self-esteem may be attributed to genetics and environment, as well as SES, with upper-middle to upper class women demonstrating higher vulnerability. Extreme obesity is also highly correlated with depression among women. Still, this does not lead to a conclusion that all obese women are depressed.

What accounts for these gender differences? Well, it's not completely understood. Some researchers have theorized that depression among the obese is highly related to the amount of prejudice and discrimination individuals receive based on their weight. Another possible pathway of obesity leading to depression is a reduction in quality of life (i.e., physical functioning, role limitations, bodily pain, etc.). Remember that physical movement and exercise can reduce depression symptoms, so reduced physical functioning can significantly contribute to depressive characteristics. You can also imagine that experiencing bodily pain on a daily basis might lead to some depressive symptoms.

These trends can begin to make some sense if you consider some societal values. Generally speaking, a greater value on physical appearance is placed on women, creating some additional pressure for women to maintain a certain ideal body type (think Barbie, or Giselle Bundchen). On the other hand, greater value may be placed on status or wealth for men. In fact, research supports this exact notion, including a study of how men and women present themselves and what they ask for in personal ads (Koestner & Wheeler, 1988). In short, in this study, males were more likely to describe their own height and professional status, and describe their preference for weight and attractiveness. Conversely, women described their own weight and had a preference for height and professional status. Two personal stories further exemplify these patterns:

1. A close personal friend enjoys telling stories from his fraternity days back in college during the late 1990s. At the time, their fraternity house consisted of approximately 75 guys, and they were in the middle of rush, which is essentially the period when new pledges are selected to begin the process of joining the fraternity. They took pictures of every pledge, mingled with them, sent them home, and then looked at each picture and discussed why, or why they shouldn't, invite the person to pledge. Toward the end of the evening, an obese freshman was the topic of discussion, and many of the fraternity brothers were getting restless and discussing what attributes he could bring to the house. At that point, one of the older brothers stood on a chair and began an epic speech about why the fraternity needed more "fat kids." The details are secondhand and hazy at best, although our friend does recall that the speech ended up with a roaring chant of "FAT KIDS! FAT KIDS! FAT KIDS!" That pledge was accepted and became a popular member of the fraternity. We don't necessarily endorse this speech or pattern of thinking, although it may force you to ask yourself if you could see this happening at a sorority house instead.

2. In the car, we were listening to a local Washington, DC radio station in early 2010. The host had seen a personal ad from a woman, and in the ad, she had noted that she wanted a man who makes "good money" as the most important quality, and looks didn't even make the list. The host brilliantly asked people to call in to discuss what they considered

"good money." The phones began to light up with hundreds of women calling, all with answers ranging from $75,000 per year to $175,000 per year. Funny enough, this was the expected salary range for someone in his or her early 20s in the middle of a serious economic downturn. When the male host challenged the female radio host about this thinking, she claimed that every woman should have goals; in this case, the goal being to find a man who made a lot of money. Again, this illustrates that men and women place different values on physical appearance in relation to other qualities.

Certainly, these stories are only meant to entertain and hardly prove a point, although they do capture a snapshot of American values or gender roles. Specifically, among males, being overweight is less likely to be viewed unfavorably, and from a women's perspective, a man's weight is not quite so critical (she is more likely to value a stable job or being 6'2"). This may help explain the complex relationship between depression and obesity among men. With women, the relationship is a bit clearer; there is more stigmatization against overweight or obese women across the board, and they are more likely to be depressed.

There also has been much debate about the temporal relationship between obesity and depression, or in other words, examining whether obesity leads to depression or whether depression leads to obesity. One could logically make a case for each; people can become depressed as a result of their obesity and resulting low self-image and discrimination. Conversely, people experiencing depression may tend to overeat and have limited activity, leading to weight gain. However, as many scientists will argue, logic and reason are great, but data are better. Sadly, the data are a bit limited, and what data are available are mixed. Some studies still suggest that depression precedes obesity in adolescents, or that obesity precedes depression in older adults. However, a recent meta-analysis[3] (Rooke & Thorsteinsson, 2008) concluded that the relationship is in fact bidirectional, meaning that one can influence the other and there is no clear pattern for the population as a whole.

Finally, it's important to note that there can be numerous moderator variables that contribute to the relationship between obesity and depression, such as having an underactive thyroid, which has been associated with both obesity and depression. Another example is childhood maltreatment as a moderator variable that forms a potential link between obesity and depression. One study in particular collected data on 4,641 middle-aged women and found that both physical and sexual abuse during childhood were associated with a twofold increase in the risk of both obesity and depression as adults (Rohde et al., 2008). This information simply serves as a reminder that the relationships between obesity and psychopathological outcomes are often quite complex.

EMBARRASSMENT, SELF-ESTEEM, AND BODY IMAGE DISSATISFACTION

Although not considered a formal diagnostic category, low body image, low self-esteem, and embarrassment can be quite debilitating. In fact, we recall a reality show titled "Beauty and the Geek," that we had watched as a guilty pleasure. The show's premise was to pair self-proclaimed male "geeks" in a house with beautiful women and to see if they can learn from each other and form relationships through a series of tasks and activities. The geeks sometimes had an edge during academic challenges, whereas the beauties had an edge during tasks requiring fashion sense, popular culture knowledge, and perhaps more importantly, confidence. During one challenge, the beauties were made up to become less attractive, and several of them had to wear "fat-suits" in a bar and try to pick up men. Despite a lifetime of confidence and self-assuredness, some of these beauties were suddenly paralyzed by their appearance and humbled by how men treated them. Even in this simple, temporary exercise, the effects of having a certain appearance had an immediate impact. The embarrassment for some goes beyond socializing in bars. Reminders of one's weight can be found when eating in restaurants, going to the beach or swimming in public, or shopping for food or clothing.

Low self-esteem or negative perceptions of one's body image are not exclusive to overweight or obese individuals. In fact, some research suggests that more than half of adolescents are not satisfied with their appearance or weight (Banitt et al., 2008). Body image dissatisfaction and dissatisfaction with weight are more significant problems among women (especially of higher SES), with 16% of *normal-weight* women reporting that they believe they are too heavy (Rahman & Berenson, 2010). In fact, body image dissatisfaction is so pervasive in adolescent girls, regardless of their weight, that low body image has been described as normal.

Interestingly, the relationship between body image and *objective* measures of obesity is not quite clear. Some research suggests that there is only a weak relationship between individuals' perceptions of their appearances and the objective reality of their appearances, and that any resulting symptoms of depression or low self-esteem are actually not a function of the degree of obesity, but of self-perception. As we described above, perception does play a large role in the psychosocial impacts of obesity. You may know of someone who you view as thin, whereas they continually comment on how heavy they are. Generally speaking, most experts agree that body image problems are often a result of weight-based teasing or stigmatization, and it's likely that overweight or obese individuals (particularly women) experience more of it than normal-weight peers.

Some research suggests that overweight or obese individuals describe themselves negatively and as having low self-confidence more often than normal-weight peers; and these same individuals describe themselves positively less often than normal-weight peers (Rimm, 2004; Strauss, 2000). Strauss (2000) also found that obese children with lower self-esteem were more likely to be sad, lonely, stressed, and nervous. As it turns out, stress causes cravings for carbohydrates (Rimm, 2004), leading to increased weight gain and the worsening of these issues.

To give you some insight into the added stressors of being an overweight child or adolescent (as if adolescence isn't difficult enough), Rimm (2004) highlighted the various concerns and worries of overweight children and adolescents, which included the following:

- Popularity and attractiveness, which was more of a concern among girls
- Clothing and not being able to find cool clothes that would fit them properly
- Bullying
- Loneliness
- Being too fat for sex
- Less optimism about the future or prospects for marriage

EATING DISORDERS

Eating disorders generally refer to a pattern of disturbances in eating behavior. Obesity and eating disorders are often thought of as opposite sides of the same coin. On the one side, you have the most commonly known eating disorders, anorexia and bulimia nervosa, both characterized by unhealthy obsessions with weight. And on the other side you have obesity. Although obesity is related to an increased risk of certain eating disorders, as we will discuss, we want to emphasize that they are very different issues. Obesity is *not* an eating disorder, and individuals who are obese do not necessarily have an eating disorder. The vast majority do not. In fact, only 2% to 5% of obese individuals meet diagnostic criteria for Binge Eating Disorder (BED; Hill, 2007).

Among the identifiable eating disorders, BED (proposed for inclusion in the 5th edition of the *DSM*) is the most prevalent among overweight and obese people. BED is characterized by a repeated pattern of:

- eating quantities of food larger than what most people would eat in a two-hour window;
- feeling out of control in relation to one's eating;
- feeling distressed as a result.

Additionally, individuals with BED may

- eat very rapidly;
- eat past the point of fullness;
- eat large amounts when not hungry;
- eat alone because they are embarrassed;
- feel depressed or guilty (American Psychiatric Association, 2010).

Probably not to your surprise though, the relationship is indirect. For example, the majority of research suggests that, compared with obese persons without BED, obese individuals with BED are more likely to report not only increased symptoms of depression but also lower self-esteem, shame, guilt, greater symptoms of borderline personality disorder, and a significantly greater lifetime prevalence of any Axis I disorder, including substance abuse and depression. These consequences can, in turn, result in more binge eating problems, and the cycle continues. Notably, more than a third of obese individuals in weight-loss treatment report problems with binge eating (Hill, 2007). Perhaps more notably, treating people for BED typically does not result in significant weight loss (Hill, 2007), adding support to the fact that BED and obesity are separate issues.

Obese individuals (particularly females and youth), or individuals who perceive themselves as overweight, are more likely to develop eating disorders such as bulimia nervosa, or to lose weight in other unhealthy (but not necessarily diagnosable) ways, such as starvation diets, smoking, induced vomiting, diet pills, and so on. Childhood obesity and parent obesity are risk factors for developing bulimia nervosa (Hill, 2007). It may be that in these households, there is an unhealthy dialogue about weight, which predisposes children to body image dissatisfaction and disturbed eating patterns later on.

An alarming fact is that children who diet tend to gain more weight than those who do not (Neumark-Sztainer et al., 2006), in part due to the cycle of highly restricted eating followed by episodes of binge eating. Another explanation is that children at risk for obesity (i.e., those with parents or siblings who are obese or overweight) may be more likely to diet, more likely to be unsuccessful, and then also more likely to go on to be overweight or obese themselves. In any case, it appears that dieting in youth is actually counterproductive. Not only does obesity place youth at risk for certain eating disorders and disturbances, but these unhealthy eating patterns can place youth at risk for obesity in the future. One important caveat is that youth enrolled in clinical weight-loss programs with health professionals do not face an increased risk of eating disorders (Butryn & Wadden, 2005). However, with more and more adolescents viewing themselves as overweight, and up to 25% of 11-year-old girls already having tried to diet at least once (Hill, 2002), the risk of restrictive and unhealthy eating behaviors shows no sign of abating.

ATTENTION DEFICIT/HYPERACTIVITY DISORDER

AD/HD has garnered an incredible amount of attention (no pun intended) in recent years, in part due to the surge in research and knowledge about how we understand individual attention, and perhaps more importantly, the recognition of how significant attention problems can wreak havoc on an individual's daily functioning. We will spare you a long, technical definition of AD/HD (also still often referred to "ADD"), although we will again remind you that to officially claim a disorder, it needs to have a significant impact on daily functioning. Certainly, many people claim, and even brag, about having "ADD moments," although those moments alone do not indicate AD/HD. We digress—how are AD/HD and obesity related?

First, let's begin with a brief review of a discussion we had earlier in the chapter. We know that obesity leads to decreases in exercise, and exercise can improve attention. Put together, we might assume that as a whole, obesity leads to less exercise and decreased attention for the population at large. Then, let's review the discussion on decreases in brain volume among obese adults in areas that affect attention. Perhaps, you're already convinced of a connection.

New research is showing a more direct link between AD/HD and obesity, with direct correlations found in several research studies for children and adults. Individuals with AD/HD tend to report more impulsive overeating and less planning of meals leading to more fast-food purchases. Further, those with AD/HD may have more difficulty keeping to a strict weight-loss program (those that include keeping food records, planning diets, preparing meals, and exercising regularly). Some have gone as far to say that for many, treating AD/HD should come before attempts to treat obesity.

All that said, no clear causal link has been determined; although we do recognize the strong association. Some have hypothesized about the causal link, however. For example, some believe that the link comes down to dopamine levels, which play a role in our brain's reward system (Campbell & Eisenberg, 2007). Simply put, the more dopamine, the better we feel. Individuals with AD/HD tend to have lower dopamine levels than their counterparts without AD/HD, and guess what a big source of dopamine can be...you guessed it—food! That, combined with poor impulse control and tendency for overeating *may* contribute to the link between AD/HD and obesity.

We have heard questions such as, "Wouldn't a hyperactive child, who tends to be, well, more active, be less likely to become obese?" Quite simply, the answer is no. As stated clearly by Holtkamp et al. (2004), "being 'hyperactive' in the sense of the *DSM-IV* diagnosis of AD/HD does not prevent the development or persistence of overweight and obesity in children" (p. 685).

SEXUAL DYSFUNCTION

Sexual problems (e.g., erectile dysfunction [ED] or impotence) can lead to significant impairments in quality of life. Conversely, a healthy sex life can lead to numerous positive outcomes, including boosting immunity, burning calories, reducing stress, reducing pain, and improving sleep, to name a few. Sadly, obesity has been identified as a risk factor for sexual dysfunction for both men and women (Esposito & Giugliano, 2005), including impotence and ED.

It's not obesity alone that leads to sexual dysfunction; it's conditions associated with obesity, such as cardiovascular disease, diabetes, and metabolic syndrome. The problem is also not permanent, as obese individuals who eventually lose weight and develop better exercise habits can experience improvements in sexual functioning.

OTHER PSYCHOPATHOLOGICAL DISORDERS

Obesity and overweight are associated with other disorders as well. For example, obesity and overweight are more prevalent among individuals with bipolar disorder, although only to a small to moderate degree. Nevertheless, obese individuals tend to experience more severe episodes than their normal-weight counterparts. Obesity and overweight are also disproportionately represented among clinical samples of individuals with schizophrenia; however, it's possible that this is due to the use of some antipsychotic medications that cause weight gain.

SUMMARY

Obese and overweight individuals are at heightened risk for a host of negative psychological, emotional, social, educational, and occupational outcomes. However, the relationship between obesity and many outcomes are quite complex and often inter-related or indirect. In fact, with regard to psychopathology, many years of research support that *most* obese individuals do not present with psychopathological disorders. Rather, higher rates of psychopathology are found among clinical samples of the obese who seek medical care. One assumption that can be made is that obese individuals experiencing severe psychological problems may seek medical treatment for obesity with the hope of decreasing their psychological symptoms.

Now that you are crystal clear on the psychosocial correlates and consequences of obesity, we will move on to the medical issues related to obesity.

NOTES

[1]The facts within this section are based on information available as of the writing of this book.

[2]Interestingly, studies seem to imply a unidirectional cause between obesity and decreases in brain volume (i.e., obesity leads to brain atrophy, perhaps due to obesity's effects on vascular functioning). However, we also consider a bidirectional relationship, where it's possible that deficits in the frontal lobes, which are responsible for delay of gratification, inhibiting impulsivity, etc., may contribute to poor food choices and therefore obesity.

[3]A meta-analysis is a systematic review of many studies that combines evidence to help determine overall conclusions and quantify the size of an effect.

REFERENCES

Adams, K., Sargent, R. G., Thompson, S. H., Richter, D., Corwin, S. J., & Rogan, T. J. (2000). A study of body weight concerns and weight control practices of 4th and 7th grade adolescents. *Ethnicity & Health, 5*(1), 79–94.

American Psychiatric Association. (2000). *Diagnostic and statistical manual of mental disorders* (4th ed.-rev.). Washington, DC: Author.

American Psychiatric Association. (2010). *DSM-5 Development.* Washington, DC: Author. Retrieved June 2, 2010, from http://www.dsm5.org/ProposedRevisions/Pages/proposedrevision.aspx?rid=372

Banitt, A. A., Kaur, H., Pulvers, K. M., Nollen, N. L., Ireland, M., & Fitzgibbon, M. L. (2008). BMI percentiles and body image discrepancy in black and white adolescents. *Obesity (Silver Spring, Md.), 16*(5), 987–991.

Bethell, C., Simpson, L., Stumbo, S., Carle, A. C., & Gombojav, N. (2010). National, state, and local disparities in childhood obesity. *Health Affairs (Project Hope), 29*(3), 347–356.

Brownell, K. D., & Napolitano, M. A. (1995). Distorting reality for children: Body size proportions of Barbie and Ken dolls. *The International Journal of Eating Disorders, 18*(3), 295–298.

Butryn, M. L., & Wadden, T. A. (2005). Treatment of overweight in children and adolescents: Does dieting increase the risk of eating disorders? *The International Journal of Eating Disorders, 37*(4), 285–293.

Campbell, B. C., & Eisenberg, D. (2007). Obesity, attention deficit-hyperactivity disorder and the dopaminergic reward system. *Collegium Antropologicum, 31*(1), 33–38.

Carpenter, K. M., Hasin, D. S., Allison, D. B., & Faith, M. S. (2000). Relationships between obesity and DSM-IV major depressive disorder, suicide ideation, and suicide attempts: Results from a general population study. *American Journal of Public Health, 90*(2), 251–257.

Christakis, N. A., & Fowler, J. H. (2007). The spread of obesity in a large social network over 32 years. *The New England Journal of Medicine, 357*(4), 370–379.

Cohen-Cole, E., & Fletcher, J. M. (2008). Is obesity contagious? Social networks vs. environmental factors in the obesity epidemic. *Journal of Health Economics, 27*(5), 1382–1387.

Cook, S. J., MacPherson, K., & Langille, D. B. (2007). Weight perception, weight control, and associated risky behaviour of adolescent girls in Nova Scotia. *Canadian Family Physician, 53*, 678–684.

Cramer, P., & Steinwert, T. (1998). Thin is good, fat is bad: How early does it begin? *Journal of Applied Developmental Psychology, 19*, 429–451.

Crosnoe, R. (2007). Gender, obesity, and education. *Sociology of Education, 80*, 241–260.

Dorsey, R. R., Eberhardt, M. S., & Ogden, C. L. (2009). Racial/ethnic differences in weight perception. *Obesity (Silver Spring, Md.), 17*(4), 790–795.

Dwivedi, G., & Dwivedi, S. (2007). Sushruta—the clinician—teacher par excellence. *Journal of Chest Diseases and Allied Sciences, 49*, 243–244.

Esposito, K., & Giugliano, D. (2005). Obesity, the metabolic syndrome, and sexual dysfunction. *International Journal of Impotence Research, 17*(5), 391–398.

Gunnell, J. J., & Ceci, S. J. (2010). When emotionality trumps reason: A study of individual processing style and juror bias. *Behavioral Sciences & the Law*, 28(6), 850–877.

He, M., & Evans, A. (2007). Are parents aware that their children are overweight or obese? Do they care? *Canadian Family Physician Médecin De Famille Canadien*, 53(9), 1493–1499.

Hill, A. J. (2002). Prevalence and demographics of dieting. In C. G. Fairburn, & K. D. Brownell (Eds.). *Eating disorders and obesity* (pp. 80–83, 2nd ed.). New York: Guilford Press.

Hill, A. J. (2007). Obesity and eating disorders. *Obesity Reviews*, 8, 151–155.

Holtkamp, K., Konrad, K., Müller, B., Heussen, N., Herpertz, S., Herpertz-Dahlmann, B., & Hebebrand, J. (2004). Overweight and obesity in children with Attention-Deficit/Hyperactivity Disorder. *International Journal of Obesity*, 28, 685–689.

Jones, L. R., Fries, E., & Danish, S. J. (2007). Gender and ethnic differences in body image and opposite sex figure preferences of rural adolescents. *Body Image*, 4(1), 103–108.

Koestner, R., & Wheeler, L. (1988). Self-presentation in personal advertisements: The influence of implicit notions of attraction and role expectations. *Journal of Social and Personal Relationships*, 5, 149–160.

Libbey, H. P., Story, M. T., Neumark-Sztainer, D. R., & Boutelle, K. N. (2008). Teasing, disordered eating behaviors, and psychological morbidities among overweight adolescents. *Obesity (Silver Spring, Md.)*, 16(Suppl. 2), S24–S29.

Lumeng, J. C., Forrest, P., Appugliese, D. P., Kaciroti, N., Corwyn, R. F., & Bradley, R. H. (2010). Weight status as a predictor of being bullied in third through sixth grades. *Pediatrics*, 125(6), e1301–e1307.

Malinauskas, B. M., Raedeke, T. D., Aeby, V. G., Smith, J. L., & Dallas, M. B. (2006). Dieting practices, weight perceptions, and body composition: A comparison of normal weight, overweight, and obese college females. *Nutrition Journal*, 5, 11.

Neumark-Sztainer, D., Falkner, N., Story, M., Perry, C., Hannan, P. J., & Mulert, S. (2002). Weight-teasing among adolescents: Correlations with weight status and disordered eating behaviors. *International Journal of Obesity and Related Metabolic Disorders: Journal of the International Association for the Study of Obesity*, 26(1), 123–131.

Neumark-Sztainer, D., Story, M., & Harris, T. (1999). Beliefs and attitudes about obesity among teachers and school health care providers working with adolescents. *Journal of Nutrition Education, 31,* 3–9.

Neumark-Sztainer, D., Wall, M., Guo, J., Story, M., Haines, J., & Eisenberg, M. (2006). Obesity, disordered eating, and eating disorders in a longitudinal study of adolescents: How do dieters fare 5 years later? *Journal of the American Dietetic Association, 106*(4), 559–568.

Peters, W. (1971a). *A class divided.* Garden City, NY: Doubleday.

Peters, W. (1971b). *The eye of the storm.* New York, NY: American Broadcasting Company.

Puhl, R., & Brownell, K. D. (2001). Bias, discrimination, and obesity. *Obesity Research, 9*(12), 788–805.

Puhl, R. M., Andreyeva, T., & Brownell, K. D. (2008). Perceptions of weight discrimination: Prevalence and comparison to race and gender discrimination in America. *International Journal of Obesity (2005), 32*(6), 992–1000.

Puhl, R. M., & Brownell, K. D. (2003). Psychosocial origins of obesity stigma: Toward changing a powerful and pervasive bias. *Obesity Reviews: An Official Journal of the International Association for the Study of Obesity, 4*(4), 213–227.

Puhl, R. M., & Heuer, C. A. (2010). Obesity stigma: Important considerations for public health. *American Journal of Public Health, 100*(6), 1019–1028.

Rahman, M., & Berenson, A. B. (2010). Self-perception of weight and its association with weight-related behaviors in young, reproductive-aged women. *Obstetrics and Gynecology, 116*(6), 1274–1280.

Raji, C. A., Ho, A. J., Parikshak, N. N., Becker, J. T., Lopez, O. L., Kuller, L. H.,…Thompson, P. M. (2010). Brain structure and obesity. *Human Brain Mapping, 31*(3), 353–364.

Rimm, S. (2004). *Rescuing the emotional lives of overweight children: What our kids go through—And how we can help.* New York, NY: Rodale Press.

Roehling, M. V. (1999). Weight-based discrimination in employment: Psychological and legal aspects. *Personnel Psychology, 52,* 969–1016.

Rohde, P., Ichikawa, L., Simon, G. E., Ludman, E. J., Linde, J. A., Jeffery, R. W., & Operskalski, B. H. (2008). Associations of child sexual and physical abuse with obesity and depression in middle-aged women. *Child Abuse & Neglect, 32*(9), 878–887.

Rooke, S. E., & Thorsteinsson, E. B. (2008). Examining the temporal relationship between depression and obesity: Meta-analylses of prospective research. *Health Psychology Review, 2,* 94–109.

Schwartz, M. B., Chambliss, H. O., Brownell, K. D., Blair, S. N., & Billington, C. (2003). Weight bias among health professionals specializing in obesity. *Obesity Research, 11*(9), 1033–1039.

Skelton, J. A., Busey, S. L., & Havens, P. L. (2006). Weight and health status of inner city African American children: Perceptions of children and their parents. *Body Image, 3*(3), 289–293.

Staffieri, J. R. (1967). A study of social stereotype of body image in children. *Journal of Personality and Social Psychology, 7*(1), 101–104.

Strauss, R. S. (2000). Childhood obesity and self-esteem. *Pediatrics, 105*(1), e15.

Stunkard, A. J., LaFleur, W. R., & Wadden, T. A. (1998). Stigmatization of obesity in medieval times: Asia and Europe. *International Journal of Obesity and Related Metabolic Disorders: Journal of the International Association for the Study of Obesity, 22*(12), 1141–1144.

Thompson, A. A. (2010). Obesity as a disability under the Americans with Disabilities Act Amendments Act and the Amendments' affect on obesity claims under the Pennsylvania Human Relations Act: Should employers anticipate a big change? *Duquesne Business Law Journal, 12,* 259–272.

Vener, A. M., Krupka, L. R., & Gerard, R. J. (1982). Overweight/obese patients: An overview. *The Practitioner, 226*(1368), 1102–1109.

Ward, M. A., Carlsson, C. M., Trivedi, M. A., Sager, M. A., & Johnson, S. C. (2005). The effect of body mass index on global brain volume in middle-aged adults: A cross sectional study. *BMC Neurology, 5,* 23.

Whitaker, K. L., Jarvis, M. J., Beeken, R. J., Boniface, D., & Wardle, J. (2010). Comparing maternal and paternal intergenerational transmission of obesity risk in a large population-based sample. *The American Journal of Clinical Nutrition, 91*(6), 1560–1567.

Wolin, K. Y., & Petrelli, J. M. (2009). *Obesity.* Santa Barbara, CA: Greenwood Publishing Group.

Xie, B., Chou, C. P., Spruijt-Metz, D., Reynolds, K., Clark, F., Palmer, P. H., Gallaher, P., Sun, P., Guo, Q., & Johnson, C. A. (2006). Weight perception and weight-related sociocultural and behavioral factors in Chinese adolescents. *Preventive Medicine, 42*(3), 229–234.

Yee, D. (2004). *Feds: Obesity raising airline fuel costs* (Associated Press). Retrieved April 17, 2011, from http://www.usatoday.com/travel/news/2004–11-05-obese-fliers_x.htm

Medical Correlates and Consequences of Obesity

This likely comes as no surprise: obesity is bad for you. The medical and physical consequences of obesity are both significant and numerous. In fact, obesity ranks as one of the most serious preventable health problems facing society today. Although not all-inclusive, this chapter will discuss the various medical problems associated with obesity among children and adults, as well as the long-term medical consequences of obesity. First, we will provide a brief medical history of obesity, which will give a context to our understanding of its medical consequences today.

MEDICAL HISTORY OF OBESITY

"The history of obesity is a history of failure" (Haslam, 2007, p. 31). Haslam made this remark in the context of a long history of awareness and knowledge of how to best manage obesity, yet a continued rise in its prevalence. Even Hippocrates, who lived around 400 BC, recognized the relationship of diet and health by commenting on the differences observed between the diets of the healthy and the diets of the sick.

Throughout the history of mankind, various methods of addressing obesity have been documented. Many of these methods mirror strategies seen today, for better or worse: binging and purging (ancient Egyptians), eating in moderation (Pythagoras, circa 500 BC, and yes the same Pythagoras from your high school geometry class), and even combining exercise with diet for optimal health (Iccus and Herodicus, circa 500–400 BC). In fact, Herodicus was censured by Plato for prolonging life by prescribing modifications to diet and activity level, rather than letting people die (Haslam, 2007).

Hippocrates and others carried on the idea of combining exercise and diet, not eating to the point of utter discomfort, and only eating—get this—to the point of satisfaction. More philosophers and physicians began recognizing that weight could be controlled by exercising and limiting food, and even limiting alcohol consumption. This knowledge carried through the centuries into modern times, leading to new research, knowledge, and innovations. For the most part, however, our basic knowledge of weight management remains fairly similar to the tenets set forth by those individuals almost 2500 years ago. When you think about our advancement in other areas (e.g., communication, space exploration, luggage with wheels), disappointment in our progress managing obesity is probably justified.

Around the 1600s and 1700s, interest began to shift from the preservation of health to the prevention of disease (Haslam, 2007). Further, in 1660, the phrase "obesity" was first documented in the literature. Physicians began to recognize the association between obesity and various other disorders or conditions, including shortness of breath, diabetes, coronary heart disease (CHD), lethargy, depression, ulcers, sleep apnea, and poor circulation (Haslam, 2007). Some physicians during the 1700s also realized that preventing obesity is easier and more effective than treatment and intervention of the obese. By 1864, the first diet plan was written, which has been likened to a forerunner of the Atkins diet (Haslam, 2007).

MEDICAL AND PHYSICAL CONSEQUENCES OF OBESITY

Mortality

What more appropriate way to open the discussion of medical consequences of overweight and obesity than talking about mortality (i.e., the increased risk of death associated with obesity)? Put simply, obesity is related to marked reductions in life expectancy (Fontaine, Redden, Wang, Westfall, & Allison, 2003) for all ethnic and racial groups, as well as for both men and women, largely due to cardiovascular disease. For years, smoking has held the title of being the leading behavioral risk factor for mortality in the United States, accounting for 18.1% of total U.S. deaths in 2000 (Mokdad, Marks, Stroup, & Gerberding, 2004). However, obesity is catching up quickly. Poor diet and physical inactivity (i.e., the things that lead to obesity) were responsible for 16.6% of total U.S. deaths in 2000 (Mokdad et al., 2004). A recent study revealed that obesity has emerged as the number one public health threat (in terms of overall disease burden), which is in part due to the overall decrease in smoking and the continued rapid increase in obesity prevalence (Jia & Lubetkin, 2010).

For most age groups, the lowest risk of mortality occurs for individuals in the normal body weight range (20–24.9 kg/m^2).

Results from the Framingham Heart Study demonstrated that adults of normal weight lived six to seven years longer than adults who were obese at age 40 (Peeters et al., 2003). Further, research has found that extreme obesity (body mass index [BMI] above 45 kg/m^2) in individuals between 20 and 30 years of age was associated with a minimum of eight years of life lost for women and 13 years of life lost for men (Fontaine et al., 2003).

The number of annual deaths attributable to obesity ranges from 111,909 (Flegal, Graubard, Williamson, & Gail, 2005), the approximate population of Ann Arbor, MI, to 414,000 (Mokdad et al., 2004), nearly the population of Cleveland, OH. You may be thinking to yourself "That's an enormous range—which one is it?" Well, it's more difficult to measure than something like death from car accidents or homicide, but the most recent analyses point to a number somewhere in the neighborhood of 299,000 to 363,000 (Flegal, Graubard, Williamson, & Gail, 2010)—or in other terms, the approximate population of Boulder, CO, to the approximate population of Tallahassee, FL.

The risk of mortality among overweight (moderate elevation in BMI, as opposed to obesity), however, has been questioned, with research showing varied results. Some studies demonstrate no increase in mortality among overweight, or even a *decreased* mortality risk when compared with normal-weight peers (e.g., Finkelstein, Brown, Wrage, Allaire, & Hoerger, 2010; Orpana et al., 2010), leading some to believe that overweight serves as a protective factor in some way. However, some studies show otherwise, leading to disagreement and controversy about the mortality risk of overweight. Some researchers have speculated that smoking may confound these results, given that smoking results in a lower BMI but an increased mortality risk. To address this theory, one study compared 186,000 adults who had never smoked and found that the mortality risk among overweight 50 to 71 year olds increased significantly when compared with those of normal weight (Adams et al., 2006). In addition, a recent study compiled data from 19 prospective studies that included 1.46 million individuals and found that overweight and obesity were associated with increases in all-cause mortality when looking only at individuals who had never smoked or been diagnosed with cancer or heart disease (Berrington de Gonzalez et al., 2000). At this point, the jury is out on mortality and moderately elevated BMI, although the science unequivocally demonstrates increased mortality risk for those in the obese range.

Interestingly, underweight is associated with greater mortality risk as well, creating a U- or J-shaped curve between BMI and mortality (Calle, Thun, Petrelli, Rodriguez, & Heath, 1999). In other words, mortality rates are higher for those with a BMI in the underweight range, then dip for normal BMI, and then rise sharply for those with a higher BMI, creating a J- or U-shaped curve, depending on the population studied. An example of a J-shaped curve can be seen in Figure 4.1.

Quality Adjusted Life Years

Some people may be familiar with a game called, "Would You Rather...?" where someone asks you to choose between two scenarios. For example, would you rather have the power of flight or invisibility? Would you rather read this book or go to the dentist? Don't answer that. Well, here's one for you—would

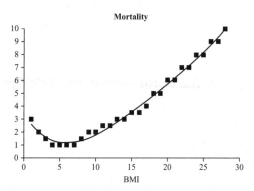

FIGURE 4.1 An example of the J- or U-shaped mortality curve.

you rather live an extra eight years at half the quality of life that you have now, or live four years in good health? Some people may be more familiar with the question "Would you rather live an extra six years but never get to eat another dessert again?" Basically, these questions are designed to get you to make tradeoffs, and your answers tell us what you value.

Aside from simply looking at statistics on mortality, a great deal of research has begun to clarify that not only do obese individuals live fewer years but also the *quality* of those years is reduced as well. Further, despite grim mortality statistics for the obese, the lives of obese individuals are extended more so than in the past due to advanced medicine (e.g., medication for diabetes or life-saving heart surgery), even though the quality of life is diminished. Researchers have found a way to measure the quality of life using the kinds of tradeoffs we discussed above (of course with some margin of error since the answers are pretty subjective), which is referred to as quality adjusted life years (QALYs). So for example, a year living with diabetes may be equivalent to three years living with cat allergies and a feline-loving roommate, or three months living in perfect health. If a year in perfect health is equal to 100, then a year of severe obesity may only count for 50 (these are just made up numbers, don't go quoting us on them). You get the idea. A recently published study determined that QALYs lost due to obesity have more than doubled from 1993 to 2008 among a sample of U.S. adults (Jia & Lubetkin, 2010). Black women emerged as having the most QALYs lost due to obesity.

Obesity and Mortality Across the Life Span

Although the relationship between BMI and mortality is well established, some research suggests that the nature and strength of this relationship are not uniform across the life span. The relationship between high BMIs and mortality weakens over the life span (Stevens et al., 1998), such that BMIs in the overweight range are actually associated with the lowest risk of mortality in older adults (Durazo-Arvizu, McGee, Cooper, Liao, & Luke, 1998; Heiat, Vaccarino, & Krumholz, 2001). As noted above, these epidemiological studies have often failed to control for confounding effects of smoking or underlying disease, which could contribute to lower body weights in older adulthood (Losonczy et al., 1995). In other words, older adults are more likely to suffer from diseases such as cancer, which can cause weight loss *and* mortality. Additionally, a survival bias may play a role, whereby individuals sensitive to the negative health consequences of obesity may have died at younger ages, resulting in older age cohorts that are more resistant to obesity-related comorbidities (National Heart, Lung, and Blood Institute, 1998). As with many other issues we have discussed, it is not clear at this point what exactly the BMI–mortality curve looks like across the life span.

Morbidity

Obesity is associated with significant increases in the risk of numerous medical and physical conditions. In fact, 85% of obese people develop some type of comorbidity throughout their lives (Reaven, 2003). The prevalence of most obesity-related comorbidities and metabolic risk factors (e.g., hypertension, diabetes, cardiovascular disease, osteoarthritis) increases with age (Klein et al., 2004; Villareal, Apovian, Kushner, & Klein, 2005; Villareal, Banks, Siener, Sinacore, & Klein, 2004).

The link between obesity and related diseases and risk factors, however, is not wholly consistent across the life span. Longitudinal studies have found that obesity is related to heightened risk of CHD, heart attacks, and cardiovascular disease mortality in older men, but not necessarily in older women (Dey & Lissner, 2003; Stevens et al., 1998). Further, obesity has been implicated as a protective factor against bone loss in older adults (Rossner, 2001), as well as contributing to reduced risk of osteoporosis and hip fracture (Felson, Zhang, Hannan, & Anderson, 1993).

Despite these exceptions, evidence supporting the link between obesity and increased morbidity and mortality continues to accrue. Aside from mortality and reduced quality of life addressed above, obesity correlates with a heightened risk of numerous health conditions, such as:

- Coronary heart and cardiovascular disease
- Hypertension, or high blood pressure
- Dyslipidemia or high cholesterol and triglycerides
- Type 2 diabetes
- Gallstones
- Metabolic syndrome
- Stroke
- Osteoarthritis and musculoskeletal problems
- Sleep apnea and other respiratory problems
- Cancer
- Frailty in older adults
- Dementia
- Complications during pregnancy
- Hot flashes

As obesity becomes much more common (and as our population ages), so do these negative health consequences. This is concerning not only for the vast number of individuals who now have to deal with these health issues but also for society at large. The costs to society of obesity and related health issues are tremendous (see Chapter 1). We will briefly provide some detail about these medical conditions.

Coronary Heart and Cardiovascular Disease

Coronary heart disease (CHD) affects approximately 14 million people in the United States and represents the leading cause of death. In fact, approximately one individual will die from a coronary event every minute. CHD is a narrowing of the blood vessels delivering blood and oxygen to the heart due to a build-up of fatty material and plaque on the artery wall. Some research suggests that overweight individuals are almost twice as likely to develop CHD as normal-weight peers, and obese individuals are approximately three times as likely to develop CHD. Importantly, with increased risk of CHD comes increased risk of dying from it (Field, Barnoya, & Colditz, 2002).

Childhood obesity is also associated with increased risk of CHD in adulthood. Obese children are 1.7 to 2.6 times as likely to develop CHD as adults when compared with normal-weight peers (Freedman, 2004), with some indication that this association is stronger among males than females (Must, Jacques, Dallal, Bajema, & Dietz, 1992). In fact, Must et al. found that even after controlling for adult weight status, the relative risk of CHD in adulthood was 2.5 for men who were obese as children, whereas childhood obesity was not related to CHD in adulthood for women.

In contrast, other studies have yielded results pointing to the importance of adult weight status in predicting CHD rather than childhood weight status. These other studies found that factors such as persistence of obesity over the lifetime, or rapid weight gain in adulthood despite being thin as a child, resulted in higher rates of cardiovascular disease or CHD in adulthood.

What these studies have in common is that BMI and CHD are positively correlated, with linear associations for age across the entire BMI distribution. Given the continued increase in childhood obesity, one could predict increased CHD among future generations of adults.

Hypertension, or High Blood Pressure

Approximately one in four Americans has high blood pressure (Field et al., 2002). Hypertension itself is related to various other medical problems, including stroke, heart failure, kidney failure, atherosclerosis, or arterial aneurysm (if you don't know what those are, they are all bad things).

As you may have guessed, obesity and weight gain are associated with hypertension. In fact, obesity or overweight accounts for two thirds of the cases of hypertension. The mechanisms responsible for this association are numerous, and some are beyond the purview of this book, although one main reason is that increased fat tissue creates more resistance to blood flow, causing the heart to have to pump blood with more pressure to circulate. Imagine trying to blow a spitball through a straw—and then imagine trying to do that with some trace amounts of strawberry jam along the sides; it's sort of like that.

Obese children's risk of hypertension is three times higher when compared with normal-weight peers (Sorof & Daniels, 2002) regardless of race, gender, and age. Given the significant increase in childhood obesity in recent history, it likely comes as no surprise that childhood hypertension is also increasing in prevalence. Further, our understanding of the scope of childhood hypertension may be misunderstood, given the significant underdiagnosis of hypertension among children and adolescents (Hansen, Gunn, & Kaelber, 2007).

Dyslipidemia or High Cholesterol and Triglycerides

Most people have never heard of dyslipidemia, although anyone who has had their cholesterol checked within the past 10 years likely has some familiarity with triglycerides and high density lipids (HDL; "good" cholesterol) and low density lipids (LDL; "bad" cholesterol). Dyslipidemia simply describes a condition marked by excessively high triglycerides and LDL, with decreased HDL. Generally speaking, obesity is associated with dyslipidemia across age ranges and gender. The presence of lipid disorders such as dyslipidemia also increases the risk of atherosclerosis, heart disease, stroke, hypertension, and even pancreatitis (are you beginning to see a pattern?).

Risk of dyslipidemia tends to be worse for those with visceral obesity, or obesity concentrated in the abdomen area, when compared with those with body fat more evenly distributed throughout the body. This is likely because fatty cells located in the central region of the body are insulin resistant and recycle fatty acids more rapidly. If you wish to know more about this process, you can do an Internet search for lipolysis. Have fun.

Type 2 Diabetes

Type 2 diabetes affects millions of individuals in the United States. According to data from the National Diabetes Information Clearinghouse (2011), type 2 diabetes is more of a predominant concern for older adults, although approximately 3,600 youth (younger than age 20 years) are newly diagnosed with type 2 diabetes annually. It is particularly rare among younger children, and more prevalent among minority populations when compared with non-Hispanic Caucasian populations. Approximately 90% of the cases of diabetes in the United States are due to obesity (Hossain, Kawar, & El Nahas, 2007).

Type 2 diabetes, put simply, describes the body's lack of insulin—and insulin is critical when metabolizing sugars and starches that the body needs for fuel. Diabetes increases the risk for blindness, kidney disease, heart disease, stroke, and is the seventh leading cause of death in the United States (Field et al., 2002). It may suddenly be clear why grandma always has an unusually large stash of sugar-free candy.

Obese and overweight individuals experience increased risk for type 2 diabetes, and even further, adults at the upper end of the healthy weight range (e.g., BMI of 24) are at some increased risk. Risk increases even more when the weight is centrally located (in the waist or abdomen). Further, even modest weight gain (11–18 pounds) from age 18 years to adulthood (age 30–55 years) results in a large increase in the risk of diabetes. If you're anything like us, you might suddenly be alarmed at how much different you looked during senior year of high school compared to now.

Gallstones

Gallstone disease remains an escalating health problem, affecting approximately 10% to 15% of the American population (more frequent among women) and represents the leading cause of hospital admissions for gastrointestinal problems (Stinton, Myers, & Shaffer, 2010). Although gallstones have a low mortality and often are asymptomatic, symptoms can often appear later in life and become increasingly more severe. Some symptoms or conditions that can result from gallstones include biliary colic (which causes severe pain and nausea), inflammation of the gallbladder or pancreas, jaundice, sepsis, gallbladder cancer, and gastrointestinal problems.

Obesity is a major risk factor for gallstones and gallstone disease, especially for those with abdominal obesity and individuals who become obese earlier in life (Stinton, Meyers, & Shaffer, 2010). Interestingly, losing weight too quickly can also lead to significant risk of developing gallstones; thus, when discussing gallstone disease, it is often recommended to lose weight more gradually (sorry "Biggest Loser"). Gallstone disease is a metabolic problem. As such, the apparent link between obesity, gallstones, cholesterol, and diabetes and insulin resistance is related to the metabolic syndrome (Stinton, Myers, & Shafter, 2010).

Metabolic Syndrome

The metabolic syndrome (MetS) is a cluster of risk factors, including high blood pressure, dyslipidemia, central/abdominal obesity, and insulin resistance. It is not a disease in and of itself, but it puts individuals at substantially higher risk for cardiovascular disease and type 2 diabetes. People with the metabolic syndrome are twice as likely to develop cardiovascular disease and five times more likely to develop diabetes than individuals without the metabolic syndrome (Alberti et al., 2009). The reason it has been identified as a syndrome is that these risk factors tend to co-occur. Largely because of the increasing prevalence of obesity, the prevalence of the metabolic syndrome has increased drastically as well. The metabolic syndrome is also being seen more frequently among children than ever before, affecting about 4% of youth (Amemiya et al., 2007). Alarmingly, 14% of overweight or obese children under 10 years of age and 21% of overweight or obese adolescents meet criteria for MetS (van Vliet et al., 2009). Some estimates have ranged as high as 30% of obese children meeting criteria for MetS (Amemiya et al. 2007).

Stroke

Excessive weight leads to increased risk of stroke. This was recently confirmed by a 19-year longitudinal study consisting of 13,549 participants, which also determined that the degree of risk varied by sex and ethnicity, with particularly higher risk for African Americans and Asian Americans (Yatsuya et al., 2010). If you're not convinced, a meta-analysis of studies with nearly a combined 2.3 million participants revealed an increasing risk of stroke with increases in weight, independent of age and lifestyle (Strazzullo et al., 2010).

Many believe that the increased risk of stroke from obesity has something to do with the fact that both obesity and stroke are also associated with high blood pressure, diabetes, and some of the other aforementioned comorbidities. Sadly, at this point, it is unclear whether a reduction in weight would lead to a reduction in stroke. (This is probably more a function of the fact that it is extremely difficult and expensive to get a large enough number of people to successfully lose weight and to follow them for the decades it would take to see a reduction in stroke risk.)

Osteoarthritis and Musculoskeletal Problems

An estimated 26 million individuals in the United Staes aged 25 years and older have osteoarthritis, a common musculoskeletal problem (Lawrence et al., 2008). Osteoarthritis is characterized by a wearing down of cartilage, a substance that allows bones to glide over each other smoothly. Without cartilage, the bones rub up against each other during physical activity, creating pain, swelling, stiffness, and loss of movement in the joints (particularly in the lower limbs among obese individuals). Given these potential impairments, not to mention the pain, osteoarthritis is associated with depression, anxiety, helplessness, reduced activity level, and occupational limitations.

Overweight adults are more than twice as likely to develop osteoarthritis when compared with their normal-weight peers. Further, obese individuals who have already developed osteoarthritis tend to experience additional physical stress due to the added strain on the joints from excess weight bearing, causing the osteoarthritis to advance more quickly.

Interestingly, recent research suggests that obesity can lead to musculoskeletal issues among children as well. One study in particular found that children aged 2 to 17 years reported more musculoskeletal and lower extremity problems (e.g., ankle and foot) than normal-weight peers, and saw the family physician more frequently for these issues (Krul, van der Wouden, Schellevis, van Suijlekom-Smit, & Koes, 2009).

Sleep Apnea and Other Respiratory Problems

Sleep apnea, which affects nearly 18 million Americans (National Sleep Foundation, 2011), describes an absence of breathing during sleep for at least 10 seconds and is often accompanied by snoring, disturbed sleep, and daytime sleepiness (not to mention an angry, cranky spouse the following day). It is estimated that the number of hospital visits due to sleep apnea among children aged 6 to 17 years has increased 436% in the past 20 years—which is largely attributed to the rapid increase in childhood obesity.

Some of the consequences of apnea, aside from sometimes waking up in the middle of night from not breathing, include hypertension, cardiac arrhythmias, arterial hypoxemia (insufficient oxygenation of the blood), accidents caused by daytime sleepiness (e.g., reduced response time while driving), and sympathetic overactivity. Obesity, hypertension, and sleep apnea are closely linked, and under certain conditions, obesity has been viewed as a causal link to sleep apnea (Poulain et al., 2006). Approximately 77% of obese adults report sleeping problems such as sleep apnea (National Sleep Foundation, 2011).

Sleep apnea, much like the other consequences of obesity, appears to exist within a self-fulfilling cycle. An overweight individual is often less motivated to exercise or remain active, and more likely to experience sleep apnea. Sleep apnea creates higher levels of fatigue during the day, making exercise even more difficult and less appealing. Such sleep difficulties contribute to weight gain as people are less likely to exercise and more likely to eat during the day to keep themselves alert.

Aside from sleep apnea, obesity also increases the risk of other respiratory problems including chronic obstructive pulmonary disease (COPD; bronchitis or emphysema making it difficult to breathe), asthma, and obesity hypoventilation syndrome, which occurs when people's short or shallow breathing results in low blood oxygen levels and high carbon dioxide levels (Poulain et al., 2006). In fact, obesity predicts chronic asthma after puberty. These breathing problems tend to result due to reduced lung volume and accumulations of fat tissue in the throat. Reductions in weight tend to directly reduce symptoms of such respiratory diseases. Similar to sleep apnea, respiratory diseases and obesity become of a self-fulfilling cycle for many due to the exercise intolerance associated with difficulties in breathing.

Cancer

Obesity increases the risk for various forms of cancer, including cancers of the endometrium (lining of the uterus), breast (postmenopausal only), ovaries, pancreas, esophagus, kidney, liver, gallbladder, and colon. Approximately 41,300 new cases of cancer were linked to obesity in 2002 in the United States, accounting for more than 3% of all new cases of cancer (Polednak, 2003). Further, another study estimated that 14% to 20% of deaths from cancer (in men and women, respectively) were due to overweight and obesity (Calle, Rodriguez, Walker-Thurmond, & Thun, 2003). The heaviest individuals face death rates from cancer as much as 52% or 62% higher for men and women, respectively, when compared with normal-weight peers. Some estimates in Europe indicate that up to 45% of new cases of cancer can be attributed to overweight or obesity (Pischon, Nothlings, & Boeing, 2008). Here, we discuss several (but not all) forms of cancer that demonstrate a conclusive relationship to overweight and obesity. Most data reported represent figures within the United Staes, although similar data can often be found in other developed countries.

Breast Cancer

Breast cancer mostly affects women, with more than 200,000 new cases of breast cancer reported in women this year (1,970 in men); further, more than 40,000 deaths were attributed to breast cancer in 2010 alone (National Cancer Institute, 2010). Strangely enough, before menopause, obesity seems to serve as a protective factor against breast cancer—obese premenopausal women are *less* likely to develop breast cancer than women of normal weight. However, after menopause, obese women have an increased risk of breast cancer compared with normal-weight peers. This is particularly true for women with visceral obesity (abdominal fat) and those with significant weight gain during adulthood. In addition, obese women are more likely to die of breast cancer than women of a healthy weight after menopause.

The increased risk of breast cancer among postmenopausal women is thought to be due to increased estrogen levels (Toniolo et al., 1995). After menopause, fat tissue becomes the primary source of estrogen, and with more fat tissue comes heavier estrogen production (50%–100% higher production in obese women) that can lead to breast tumors (Huang et al., 1997). Higher death rates are in part due to the later diagnosis in obese women as recognition becomes more difficult with increased weight.

Endometrial (Uterine) Cancer

More than 43,000 new cases of endometrial cancer were reported in 2010, and nearly 8,000 deaths were attributed to it (National Cancer Institute, 2010). Obesity has been linked to up to 40% of cases of uterine cancer (Bergström, Pisani, Tenet, Wolk, & Adami, 2001), and the risk of developing uterine cancer is significantly increased among obese women. In fact, the risk is increased up to four times, regardless of menopause status (National Cancer Institute, 2004; Vainio & Bianchini, 2002).

Colon Cancer

Approximately 103,000 new cases of colon cancer were reported in 2010 (National Cancer Institute, 2010). Obesity increases the risk of colon cancer, although this appears to be more significant for men, for individuals who engage in little to no physical activity, and for those with more abdominal fat. Now, recall that an elevated BMI combined with increased estrogen levels (from fat tissue) were believed to play a role in breast cancer. Well, estrogen appears to be a protective factor against colon cancer for women in general. The picture is complicated, however; a high BMI appears to put women at greater risk of colon cancer if they are taking estrogens whereas for women not taking hormones, a high BMI does not increase their risk for colon cancer (Slattery, Ballard-Barbash, Edwards, Caan, & Potter, 2003).

It is thought that obesity contributes to an increased risk of colon cancer by affecting growth hormones such as insulin and insulin-like growth factors (Slattery et al., 2003).

However, there is hope; one study (that included some women taking postmenopausal hormones) found that physically active women had significantly reduced their risk of colon cancer when compared with nonactive women (Martinez et al., 1997).

Kidney Cancer

Overweight and obesity have been linked to kidney cancer, specifically renal cell cancer, across a range of studies. The National Cancer Institute estimates there were nearly 60,000 new cases of renal cell cancer in 2010 alone, with approximately 13,000 deaths from it. One study conducted a summary analysis of all studies exploring this relationship between 1966 and 1998, and identified an equally strong increase in the risk of renal cell cancer among men and women with elevated BMI (Bergström et al., 2001). This particular study attempted to clear up confusion about the role of gender and renal cell cancer risk; women with a high BMI consistently demonstrated increased risk, whereas the risk for men with a high BMI was less clear. Based on their meta-analysis, they estimated that 27% to 29% of all cases of renal cell cancer in the United States were due to overweight or obesity for men and women, respectively.

Esophagus and Stomach Cancer

Overweight and obesity lead to an increased risk of esophageal cancer, with several studies suggesting the risk to be double that of normal-weight peers (National Cancer Institute, 2004). For those who don't recall from middle-school science class, the esophagus is the muscular tube that passes food from the mouth to the stomach, and allows kids to debunk the myth that you can't eat while standing upside down. There were an estimated 16,640 new cases of esophageal cancer in 2010, with 14,500 deaths from it (National Cancer Institute, 2010). The incidence has increased approximately 350% in the past three decades, which some have attributed to the increased prevalence of obesity. A smaller (yet significant) increase in the risk of gastric cardia cancer (a type of stomach cancer) has also been found (Chow et al., 1998). It's still unclear why or how obesity and overweight increase the risk of these types of cancer.

Pancreatic Cancer

There were approximately 43,000 new cases of pancreatic cancer in 2010, with nearly 37,000 deaths attributed to it (National Cancer Institute, 2010). Whereas previous research has been somewhat inconclusive about the relationship between obesity and pancreatic cancer, more recent research has confirmed a significant association. Further, the age of weight gain and maintenance of excess body weight affects both the age of onset and prognosis of pancreatic cancer (Li et al., 2009). Among those who are severely obese, the risk is increased by 45% (Stolzenberg-Solomon et al., 2008). Given a survival rate for those with pancreatic cancer of less than 5%, this association is particularly alarming.

Gallbladder Cancer

The National Cancer Institute reported 9,670 new cases of gallbladder cancer in 2010, with 3,320 deaths attributed to it. Gallbladder cancer, like pancreatic cancer, has a high mortality rate, with a five-year survival rate of less than 10%. Previous research had found associations between obesity and gallbladder cancer, although there did not appear to be enough evidence to draw conclusions. However, a recent meta-analysis (Larsson & Wolk, 2007) revealed an increase in risk of 15% for overweight and a 66% increase for obese people when compared with those of normal weight. The association between BMI and gallbladder cancer was stronger for women than men.

Ovarian Cancer

There were approximately 22,000 new cases of ovarian cancer in 2010, with nearly 14,000 deaths estimated to result from it (National Cancer Institute, 2010). Ovarian cancer has a five-year survival rate of only 37%. A recent analysis of nearly 95,000 women found an 80% increased risk of ovarian cancer among obese women who had never taken estrogens after menopause (Leitzmann et al., 2009). Conversely, for those taking estrogens, no association was found.

Frailty in Older Adults

Frailty among older adults can be defined as "a syndrome of physical vulnerability characterized by multisystem dysfunction and lack of physiological reserve" (Blaum, Xue, Michelon, Semba, & Fried, 2005, p. 927), and is associated with various disabilities and limitations in functioning. Obesity is significantly associated with frailty among older adults, which is presumed to be caused by lower muscle quality and reduced muscle mass. Frailty caused by obesity can lead to decreased quality of life, which again would lead one to believe that weight loss is an optimal option. However, this particular association presents with its own challenges given that rapid weight loss can lead to other issues among this population. Specifically, older individuals tend to have lower bone mass density, which increases risk of fractures. Rapid weight loss leads to decreased bone mass— and obese older adults tend to actually have greater bone mass than their nonobese peers (Villareal et al., 2004). Thus, there appear to be some minimal benefits of overweight or obesity among older adults.

Dementia

Dementia affects up to 10% of individuals aged 65 years or older, although the relationship between obesity and dementia has remained inconclusive for many years. However, a recent meta-analysis revealed an independent, U-shaped relationship between dementia and obesity, with associations found between dementia and both underweight and obesity (Beydoun, Beydoun, & Wang, 2008). The associations were only moderate, however, and not apparent for overweight. Approximately 21% of all cases of Alzheimer's disease (a form of dementia) in the United States were attributed to obesity, and the relative risk of Alzheimer's was slightly stronger among obese women when compared with obese men. Vascular dementia was slightly more apparent among those with abdominal obesity and among obese men compared to women.

Complications During Pregnancy

Various complications can result from maternal obesity during pregnancy for both the mother and child, including gestational diabetes; low Apgar[1] scores; longer deliveries; increased Cesarean delivery rates; increased preterm births; postpartum infection; increased risk that the child will become obese or develop type 2 diabetes; increased risk of newborns with excessive birth weight or perinatal death, neural tube, and other birth defects; hypertensive disorders; and thromboembolic disorders. Despite these concerns, obesity rates among pregnant women have been cited as high as 38.3% (Galtier-Dereure, Boegner, & Bringer, 2000), a figure that has increased by approximately 70% from 1993 to 2003 (Kim, Dietz, England, Morrow, & Callaghan, 2007).

Neural Tube and Other Defects

A meta-analysis (Stothard, Tennant, Bell, & Rankin, 2009) revealed that higher than recommended maternal weight during pregnancy led to increased risk of neural tube defects (including spina bifida), cardiovascular/heart defects, cleft palate, hydrocephaly (build-up of spinal fluid in the brain that can compress and lead to brain damage), limb reduction (abnormalities in the development of limbs), and anorectal atresia (obstructed rectal opening). Increased risk was also seen for neural tube defects that could alter the development of the brain, including anencephaly, which leads to absence of large parts of the brain, skull, or scalp.

Hypertensive Disorders

Among obese pregnant women, the risk of hypertension is significantly higher when compared with normal-weight peers (2.2–21.4 times higher); as is the risk of preeclampsia (1.2–9.7 times higher; Galteir-Dereure et al., 2000). For good measure, preeclampsia is a condition characterized by high blood pressure, swelling, and protein in the urine that develops during pregnancy, which can lead to decreased blood flow to the baby and increased risk for seizure or stroke for the mother.

Thromboembolic Disorders (Blood Clots)

Obese pregnant women have a slightly higher risk of developing thromboembolic disorder, which is the leading cause of death among pregnant women in the United States, and is characterized by blood clots that can lead to blocked arteries. Unfortunately, giving birth via Cesarean section increases the chance of developing a blood clot and dying from it, and as noted above, obesity during pregnancy leads to increased chance of requiring a Cesarean section delivery.

Hot Flashes

Women going through menopause experience a number of symptoms, one of which includes hot flashes that lead to uncomfortable sweating and flushing. Women with higher BMIs experience more hot flashes, and women who lost weight had significant reductions in hot flashes (Huang et al., 2010).

SUMMARY

In this chapter, we have presented information on a smattering of obesity-related medical issues. There are hundreds more that we could have discussed (e.g., nonalcoholic fatty liver disease, inflammation, polycystic ovary syndrome, kidney disease), but we wanted to keep this book under 2,000 pages.

One issue that we did not discuss is whether it is obesity that is causing a medical problem, or diet, or physical inactivity. Poor diet and physical inactivity alone have negative effects on health. These behaviors also lead to, and perpetuate, obesity. So it is very difficult to tease apart what is due to obesity, what is due to diet, and what is due to inactivity. Suffice it to say that all three go hand-in-hand to create health problems. Take-home message: obesity is bad for your health. Very bad, in many, many different ways.

NOTE

[1]Apgar scores are given to a newborn immediately after delivery to evaluate health and physical condition. The score is derived from assessing five areas: Activity and muscle tone, Pulse and heart rate, Grimace response or reflexes, Appearance (skin color), and Respiration. Each area can be scored either 0, 1, or 2, with 2 being the best score, and a possible total score of 10. Low Apgar scores may indicate mild to significant health problems in newborns.

REFERENCES

Adams, K. F., Schatzkin, A., Harris, T. B., Kipnis, V., Mouw, T., Ballard-Barbash, R., ... Leitzmann, M. F. (2006). Overweight, obesity, and mortality in a large prospective cohort of persons 50 to 71 years old. *The New England Journal of Medicine, 355*(8), 763–778.

Alberti, K. G., Eckel, R. H., Grundy, S. M., Zimmet, P. Z., Cleeman, J. I., Donato, K. A., ... Smith, S. C. (2009). Harmonizing the metabolic syndrome. *Circulation, 120*, 1640–1645.

Amemiya, S., Dobashi, K., Urakami, T., Sugihara, S., Ohzeki, T., & Tajima, N. (2007). Metabolic syndrome in youths. *Pediatric Diabetes, 8*(Suppl. 9), 48–54.

Bergström, A., Hsieh, C. C., Lindblad, P., Lu, C. M., Cook, N. R., & Wolk, A. (2001). Obesity and renal cell cancer–a quantitative review. *British Journal of Cancer, 85*(7), 984–990.

Bergström, A., Pisani, P., Tenet, V., Wolk, A., & Adami, H. O. (2001). Overweight as an avoidable cause of cancer in Europe. *International Journal of Cancer, 91*(3), 421–430.

Berrington de Gonzalez, A., Hartage, P., Cerhan, J. R., Flint, A. J., Hannan, L., MacInnis, R. J.,...Thun, M. J. (2000). Body-mass index and mortality among 1.46 million white adults. *The New England Journal of Medicine, 363,* 2211–2219.

Beydoun, M. A., Beydoun, H. A., & Wang, Y. (2008). Obesity and central obesity as risk factors for incident dementia and its subtypes: A systematic review and meta-analysis. *Obesity Reviews, 9*(3), 204–218.

Blaum, C. S., Xue, Q. L., Michelon, E., Semba, R. D., & Fried, L. P. (2005). The association between obesity and the frailty syndrome in older women: The Women's Health and Aging Studies. *Journal of the American Geriatrics Society, 53*(6), 927–934.

Calle, E. E., Rodriguez, C., Walker-Thurmond, K., & Thun, M. J. (2003). Overweight, obesity, and mortality from cancer in a prospectively studied cohort of U.S. adults. *New England Journal of Medicine, 348*(17), 1625–1638.

Calle, E. E., Thun, M. J., Petrelli, J. M., Rodriguez, C., & Heath, C. W. (1999). Body-mass index and mortality in a prospective cohort of U.S. adults. *New England Journal of Medicine, 341*(15), 1097–1105.

Chow, W. H., Blot, W. J., Vaughan, T. L., Risch, H. A., Gammon, M. D., Stanford, J. L.,...Fraumeni, J. F. (1998). Body mass index and risk of adenocarcinomas of the esophagus and gastric cardia. *Journal of the National Cancer Institute, 90*(2), 150–155.

Dey, D. K., & Lissner, L. (2003). Obesity in 70-year-old subjects as a risk factor for 15-year coronary heart disease incidence. *Obesity Research, 11*(7), 817–827.

Durazo-Arvizu, R. A., McGee, D. L., Cooper, R. S., Liao, Y., & Luke, A. (1998). Mortality and optimal body mass index in a sample of the US population. *American Journal of Epidemiology, 147*(8), 739–749.

Felson, D. T., Zhang, Y., Hannan, M. T., & Anderson, J. J. (1993). Effects of weight and body mass index on bone mineral density in men and women: The Framingham study. *Journal of Bone and Mineral Research, 8*(5), 567–573.

Field, A. E., Barnoya, J., & Colditz, G. A. (2002). Epidemiology and health and economic consequences of obesity. In T. A. Wadden & A. J. Stunkard (Eds.), *Handbook of obesity treatment* (pp. 3–18). New York, NY: The Guilford Press.

Finkelstein, E. A., Brown, D. S., Wrage, L. A., Allaire, B. T., & Hoerger, T. J. (2010). Individual and aggregate years-of-life-lost associated with overweight and obesity. *Obesity (Silver Spring, Md.), 18*(2), 333–339.

Flegal, K. M., Graubard, B. I., Williamson, D. F., & Gail, M. H. (2005). Excess deaths associated with underweight, overweight, and obesity. *Journal of the American Medical Association, 293*(15), 1861–1867.

Flegal, K. M., Graubard, B. I., Williamson, D. F., & Gail, M. H. (2010). Sources of differences in estimates of obesity-associated deaths from first National Health and Nutrition Examination Survey (NHANES I) hazard ratios. *American Journal of Clinical Nutrition, 91*(3), 519–527.

Fontaine, K. R., Redden, D. T., Wang, C., Westfall, A. O., & Allison, D. B. (2003). Years of life lost due to obesity. *Journal of the American Medical Association, 289*(2), 187–193.

Freedman, D. S. (2004). Childhood obesity and coronary heart disease. In W. Kiess, C. Marcus, & M. Wabitsch (Eds.), *Obesity in childhood and adolescence* (pp. 160–169). Basel, Switzerland: Karger.

Galtier-Dereure, F., Boegner, C., & Bringer, J. (2000). Obesity and pregnancy: Complications and cost. *The American Journal of Clinical Nutrition, 71*(5 Suppl), 1242S–1248S.

Hansen, M. L., Gunn, P. W., & Kaelber, D. C. (2007). Underdiagnosis of hypertension in children and adolescents. *Journal of the American Medical Association, 298*(8), 874–879.

Haslam, D. (2007). Obesity: A medical history. *Obesity Reviews, 8*(Suppl. 1), 31–36.

Heiat, A., Vaccarino, V., & Krumholz, H. M. (2001). An evidence-based assessment of federal guidelines for overweight and obesity as they apply to elderly persons. *Archives of Internal Medicine, 161*(9), 1194–1203.

Hossain, P., Kawar, B., & El Nahas, M. (2007). Obesity and diabetes in the developing world–a growing challenge. *The New England Journal of Medicine, 356*(3), 213–215.

Huang, A. J., Subak, L. L., Wing, R., West, D. S., Hernandez, A. L., Macer, J., & Grady, D.; Program to Reduce Incontinence by Diet and Exercise Investigators. (2010). An intensive behavioral weight loss intervention and hot flushes in women. *Archives of Internal Medicine, 170*(13), 1161–1167.

Huang, Z., Hankinson, S. E., Colditz, G. A., Stampfer, M. J., Hunter, D. J., Manson, J. E.,...Willett, W. C. (1997). Dual effects of weight and weight gain on breast cancer risk. *Journal of the American Medical Association, 278*(17), 1407–1411.

Jia, H., & Lubetkin, E. I. (2010). Obesity-related quality-adjusted life years lost in the U.S. from 1993 to 2008. *American Journal of Preventive Medicine, 39*(3), 220–227.

Kim, S. Y., Dietz, P. M., England, L., Morrow, B., & Callaghan, W. M. (2007). Trends in pre-pregnancy obesity in nine states, 1993–2003. *Obesity (Silver Spring, Md.), 15*(4), 986–993.

Klein, S., Burke, L. E., Bray, G. A., Blair, S., Allison, D. B., Pi-Sunyer, X.,...Eckel, R. H. (2004). Clinical implications of obesity with specific focus on cardiovascular disease: A statement for professionals from the American Heart Association Council on Nutrition, Physical Activity, and Metabolism: Endorsed by the American College of Cardiology Foundation. *Circulation, 110*(18), 2952–2967.

Krul, M., van der Wouden, J. C., Schellevis, F. G., van Suijlekom-Smit, L. W., & Koes, B. W. (2009). Musculoskeletal problems in overweight and obese children. *Annals of Family Medicine, 7*(4), 352–356.

Larsson, S. C., & Wolk, A. (2007). Obesity and the risk of gallbladder cancer: A meta-analysis. *British Journal of Cancer, 96*(9), 1457–1461.

Lawrence, R. C., Felson, D. T., Helmick, C. G., Arnold, L. M., Choi, H., Deyo, R. A.,...Wolfe, F. (2008). Estimates of the prevalence of arthritis and other rheumatic conditions in the United States. Part II. *Arthritis and Rheumatism, 58*(1), 26–35.

Leitzmann, M. F., Koebnick, C., Danforth, K. N., Brinton, L. A., Moore, S. C., Hollenbeck, A. R.,...Lacey, J. V. (2009). Body mass index and risk of ovarian cancer. *Cancer, 115*(4), 812–822.

Li, D., Morris, J. S., Liu, J., Hassan, M. M., Day, R. S., Bondy, M. L., & Abbruzzese, J. L. (2009). Body mass index and risk, age of onset, and survival in patients with pancreatic cancer. *Journal of the American Medical Association, 301*(24), 2553–2562.

Losonczy, K. G., Harris, T. B., Cornoni-Huntley, J., Simonsick, E. M., Wallace, R. B., Cook, N. R.,…Blazer, D. G. (1995). Does weight loss from middle age to old age explain the inverse weight mortality relation in old age? *American Journal of Epidemiology, 141*(4), 312–321.

Martínez, M. E., Giovannucci, E., Spiegelman, D., Hunter, D. J., Willett, W. C., & Colditz, G. A. (1997). Leisure-time physical activity, body size, and colon cancer in women. Nurses' Health Study Research Group. *Journal of the National Cancer Institute, 89*(13), 948–955.

Mokdad, A. H., Marks, J. S., Stroup, D. F., & Gerberding, J. L. (2004). Actual causes of death in the United States, 2000. *Journal of the American Medical Association, 291*(10), 1238–1245.

Must, A., Jacques, P. F., Dallal, G. E., Bajema, C. J., & Dietz, W. H. (1992). Long-term morbidity and mortality of overweight adolescents. A follow-up of the Harvard Growth Study of 1922 to 1935. *The New England Journal of Medicine, 327*(19), 1350–1355.

National Cancer Institute. (2004). *Obesity and cancer: Questions and answers.* Retrieved November 14, 2010, from www.cancer.gov/cancertopics/factsheet/Risk/obesity#r4

National Cancer Institute. (2010). *Types of cancer.* Retrieved December 12, 2010, from http://www.cancer.gov/

National Diabetes Information Clearinghouse. (2011) *National Diabetes Statistics, 2011.* Retrieved July 20, 2011 from http://diabetes.niddk.nih.gov/dm/pubs/statistics

National Heart, Lung, and Blood Institute. (1998) Clinical guidelines on the identification, evaluation, and treatment of overweight and obesity in adults: The evidence report. *Obesity Research, 6,* 51S–209S.

National Sleep Foundation. (2011) *Sleep apnea and sleep.* Retrieved July 20, 2011, from http://www.sleepfoundation.org/article/sleep-related-problems/obstructive-sleep-apnea-and-sleep

Orpana, H. M., Berthelot, J. M., Kaplan, M. S., Feeny, D. H., McFarland, B., & Ross, N. A. (2010). BMI and mortality: Rresults from a national longitudinal study of Canadian adults. *Obesity (Silver Spring, Md.), 18*(1), 214–218.

Peeters, A., Barendregt, J. J., Willekens, F., Mackenbach, J. P., Al Mamun, A., & Bonneux, L. (2003). Obesity in adulthood and its consequences for life expectancy: A life-table analysis. *Annals of Internal Medicine, 138*(1), 24–32.

Pischon, T., Nöthlings, U., & Boeing, H. (2008). Obesity and cancer. *The Proceedings of the Nutrition Society, 67*(2), 128–145.

Polednak, A. P. (2003). Trends in incidence rates for obesity-associated cancers in the US. *Cancer Detection and Prevention, 27*(6), 415–421.

Poulain, M., Doucet, M., Major, G. C., Drapeau, V., Sériès, F., Boulet, L. P.,...Maltais, F. (2006). The effect of obesity on chronic respiratory diseases: Pathophysiology and therapeutic strategies. *Canadian Medical Association Journal, 174*(9), 1293–1299.

Reaven, G. M. (2003). Importance of identifying the overweight patient who will benefit the most by losing weight. *Annals of Internal Medicine, 138*(5), 420–423.

Rössner, S. (2001). Obesity in the elderly—a future matter of concern? *Obesity Reviews, 2*(3), 183–188.

Slattery, M. L., Ballard-Barbash, R., Edwards, S., Caan, B. J., & Potter, J. D. (2003). Body mass index and colon cancer: An evaluation of the modifying effects of estrogen (United States). *Cancer Causes & Control, 14*(1), 75–84.

Sorof, J., & Daniels, S. (2002). Obesity hypertension in children: A problem of epidemic proportions. *Hypertension, 40*(4), 441–447.

Stevens, J., Cai, J., Pamuk, E. R., Williamson, D. F., Thun, M. J., & Wood, J. L. (1998). The effect of age on the association between body-mass index and mortality. *The New England Journal of Medicine, 338*(1), 1–7.

Stinton, L. M., Myers, R. P., & Shaffer, E. A. (2010). Epidemiology of gallstones. *Gastroenterology Clinics of North America, 39*(2), 157–69, vii.

Stolzenberg-Solomon, R. Z., Adams, K., Leitzmann, M., Schairer, C., Michaud, D. S., Hollenbeck, A.,...Silverman, D. T. (2008). Adiposity, physical activity, and pancreatic cancer in the National Institutes of Health-AARP Diet and Health Cohort. *American Journal of Epidemiology, 167*(5), 586–597.

Stothard, K. J., Tennant, P. W., Bell, R., & Rankin, J. (2009). Maternal overweight and obesity and the risk of congenital anomalies: A systematic review and meta-analysis. *Journal of the American Medical Association, 301*(6), 636–650.

Strazzullo, P., D'Elia, L., Cairella, G., Garbagnati, F., Cappuccio, F. P., & Scalfi, L. (2010). Excess body weight and incidence of stroke: Meta-analysis of prospective studies with 2 million participants. *Stroke; a Journal of Cerebral Circulation, 41*(5), e418–e426.

Toniolo, P. G., Levitz, M., Zeleniuch-Jacquotte, A., Banerjee, S., Koenig, K. L., Shore, R. E., . . . Pasternack, B. S. (1995). A prospective study of endogenous estrogens and breast cancer in postmenopausal women. *Journal of the National Cancer Institute, 87*(3), 190–197.

Vainio, H., & Bianchini, F. (2002). *IARC handbooks of cancer prevention. Volume 6: Weight control and physical activity.* Lyon, France: IARC Press.

van Vliet, M., von Rosenstiel, I. A., Schindhelm, R. K., Brandjes, D. P., Beijnen, J. H., & Diamant, M. (2009). Identifying the metabolic syndrome in obese children and adolescents: Do age and definition matter? *Current Clinical Pharmacology, 4*(3), 233–238.

Villareal, D. T., Apovian, C. M., Kushner, R. F., & Klein, S. (2005). Obesity in older adults: Technical review and position statement of the American Society for Nutrition and NAASO, The Obesity Society. *The American Journal of Clinical Nutrition, 82*(5), 923–934.

Villareal, D. T., Banks, M., Siener, C., Sinacore, D. R., & Klein, S. (2004). Physical frailty and body composition in obese elderly men and women. *Obesity Research, 12*(6), 913–920.

Yatsuya, H., Folsom, A. R., Yamagishi, K., North, K. E., Brancati, F. L., & Stevens, J. (2010). Race- and sex-specific associations of obesity measures with ischemic stroke incidence in the Atherosclerosis Risk in Communities (ARIC) study. *Stroke; a Journal of Cerebral Circulation, 41*(3), 417–425.

Current Treatments for Obesity

I f you have read this far and plan to continue reading, well done. It's quite a feat to have read so much dire news and continue to stay the course. Thus far, we have identified obesity, its causes, and the myriad consequences associated with it (mostly negative). Naturally, the next question is, "ok...now what?" And away we go.

THE PROBLEM IS NOT KNOWING THE PROBLEM

Albert Einstein once said, "If I had only one hour to save the world, I would spend fifty-five minutes defining the problem, and only five minutes finding the solution." That would make for an intense hour, to be sure, but we share this quote because it draws attention to the need to first identify a problem prior to solving it. This is the reason why car mechanics charge so much just for an inspection; identifying the problem is often more than half the battle. The first part of this book demonstrates that, as a society, we have great awareness of the problem at large. But how do people fare at identifying whether they have a personal problem with overweight or obesity? [Spoiler alert: not well]

You would think that it would be relatively easy to figure out if you are overweight or obese; about as easy as owning a mirror and looking into one, or stepping on a scale, or using a body mass index (BMI) calculator on the Internet, or assessing tight-fitting clothes that used to fit comfortably. After all, weight is a common topic in the news, on popular television (TV) shows, and in commercials, and therefore remains in the front of many of our minds. Yet a shockingly high number of people incorrectly categorize their own weight status. Those of normal weight often think they are overweight, and those who are obese or overweight often think that their weights are perfectly normal. Even further, the accuracy of these perceptions has decreased over time (Johnson-Taylor, Fisher, Hubbard, Starke-Reed, & Eggers, 2008). When you ask people to categorize their own weight as normal, overweight, or obese, about 32% of normal-weight adults get the answer wrong, 38% of overweight people get the answer wrong, and 8% of obese people get the answer wrong (Dorsey, Eberhardt, & Ogden, 2009). Men are more likely to misperceive their weight status, as are African Americans, Hispanic Americans, and individuals with lower levels of education (Dorsey et al., 2009). Given that the first step in solving any problem is realizing that a problem exists, these numbers are bad news.

When it comes to children, we are even worse at identifying those who are overweight or obese. One study found that only 61% of parents correctly identified the weight status of their children (Huang et al., 2007). Even pediatricians get it wrong; overweight or obese children are not recognized or documented as having high BMIs by their primary doctor more than half the time (Benson, Baer, & Kaelber, 2009). Further, only 20% to 50% of overweight children are medically diagnosed, and even fewer get treatment (Benson et al., 2009; Dorsey, Wells, Krumholz, & Concato, 2005; Louthan et al., 2005). We're no Einsteins, but it seems that we as a society may collectively set ourselves up for failure with such a lackluster job at identifying overweight and obesity on an individual level.

WHAT ABOUT THOSE WHO KNOW THE PROBLEM?

Despite many people wrongly identifying whether they are of normal weight, are overweight, or obese, the majority of adults do correctly recognize their own weight status. Those identifying as overweight or obese often attempt to lose weight in some way or another. About half of overweight American adults try to lose weight in any given year, and about two thirds of obese adults report dieting (Baradel et al., 2009). Approximately 60% to 65% attempt to lose weight by consuming fewer calories (dieting); 61% to upwards of 80% increase physical activity levels (exercise), and 35% to upward of 50% report using both strategies (Baradel et al., 2009; Weiss, Galuska, Khan, & Serdula, 2006). Recall from Chapter 2 that although exercise plays a prominent role in weight status, food choices and eating behavior appear to be better targets for long-lasting improvements in weight between the two. Later in the chapter, we will discuss some of the various diets that some individuals attempt and how effective they are (it's nice to have things to look forward to).

WHO ATTEMPTS WEIGHT LOSS?

Women are more likely to report dieting than men, women try to lose weight at lower BMIs than men do, and women are generally less satisfied with their weight (Andreyeva, Long, Henderson, & Grode, 2010). This may not be particularly surprising, given the pressures women face to meet a standard of appearance and our previous mention that many females at an early age are already dieting. This also coincides with women consistently identifying themselves as overweight or obese more commonly than men across each BMI category, even if they are normal weight (Lemon, Rosal, Zapka, Borg, & Andersen, 2009).

Those with low levels of education are less likely to try to lose weight (even though they have higher BMIs), and African Americans are also less likely to attempt weight loss than Caucasians (Andreyeva et al., 2010). In addition, women aged 60 years and older are less likely to attempt weight loss than women aged 20 to 29 years (Weiss et al., 2006). There are numerous possible reasons for these trends, including the strength of societal pressure to be thin (or even normal weight) as well as motivation for weight loss.

MOTIVATION

One recommendation made by the National Heart, Lung, and Blood Institute Obesity Education Initiative (NHLBI, 2000) recommends that physicians assess an individual's motivation to lose weight prior to engaging in certain weight-loss treatments. This evaluation of motivation should include assessing why someone wants to lose weight, the success (or failure) of previous attempts to lose weight, support from others, knowledge of potential risks, attitudes toward physical activity, time availability, and financial barriers, if any. They make this recommendation given the extreme commitment required for significant and sustained weight loss. Thus, it seems that if certain groups of people continue to feel that they do not require weight-loss treatment and have low motivation to do so, they likely will not receive it.

GREAT EXPECTATIONS

Generally speaking, any new endeavor can lead to a discrepancy between our expectations and reality. We had a friend who tried to learn the guitar with the expectation of playing John Mayer songs within the first six months, although anyone who has ever learned an instrument knows this is not a realistic goal. Even after a few months of having learned only one chord, this friend still held on to this lofty goal. The issue with not meeting expectations is that it can lead to frustration, disappointment, and often giving up completely (just check out how full the gym is January 2nd, and then again on February 2nd). In this way, expectations also seem to play a role in weight loss. And in case you were curious, our friend quit the guitar.

Obese individuals rarely go in to a weight-loss program expecting to lose only a few pounds. They want a substantial change, naturally. As it turns out, most individuals engaging in weight-loss programs expect to lose 25% to 30% of their initial weight (Wadden et al., 2003). Unfortunately, as you will see below, even the best programs with the best outcomes lead to an average 5% to 10% weight loss—a clear disconnect between expectations and reality.

Wadden and colleagues (2003) found that even when informing obese individuals entering a weight-loss program that they can only expect to lose 5% to 15% of weight, participants still expected a 25% weight loss, which some patients have viewed as the minimum "acceptable" amount to lose. Perhaps this is one reason for attrition rates in weight-loss programs; it's a lot of work for what is perceived as a minimal reward.

TREATING OBESITY

Aside from the main categories listed above (e.g., dieting, exercise, combination), various other strategies have been used that will be reviewed throughout this chapter, including use of prescription or over-the-counter (OTC) medication, behavior modification, surgery, various diet products or formulas, taking laxatives, inducing vomiting, commercial weight-loss programs, the list goes on. Americans spend nearly $60 billion each year on weight loss and diet products (Marketdata Enterprises, Inc., 2009). Unfortunately, it seems that this money might be better spent elsewhere, as our billions worth of diet products have not resulted in lower levels of obesity across our society.

Generally speaking, there are various levels of intensity for obesity treatment. Self-initiated diets and commercial programs (e.g., Weight Watchers, low-fat diets) are typically the first step, and individuals may cycle through dozens (even hundreds) of these diets before seeking more intensive treatments. Lifestyle or behavior modification programs are typically the next line of defense, which may include modifying eating behavior or dieting, exercise, and modifying other behaviors under professional guidance (i.e., a dietician, psychologist, etc.). The third level of intensity consists of medical treatment, such as prescription medication, or a combination of lifestyle modification and medication. Finally, surgery is often a last resort for treatment for severely obese individuals with comorbidities. Unfortunately, "bariatric surgery appears to be the only reliable method of sustaining weight losses of 20% or more of initial weight" (Tsai & Wadden, 2006; p. 1289). In revisiting the issue of weight-loss expectations, it seems that surgery is the only treatment that would allow obese individuals to meet their weight-loss goals. Some promising results also have been found in some studies that combine dietary, behavioral, and physical activity interventions, and this follows the recommendations of the National

Heart, Lung, and Blood Institute and the North American Association for the Study of Obesity. However, the long-term effects are questionable, particularly without close monitoring and adherence to the programs beyond the first year.

SELF-INITIATED DIETS, BEHAVIOR MODIFICATION, AND LIFESTYLE CHANGES

Behavioral or lifestyle weight-loss treatments seek to modify eating and activity patterns through a variety of strategies. This can include dieting, physical activity, behavior modification (e.g., through counseling or self-monitoring), and other cognitive-behavioral strategies designed to aid individuals in developing a set of skills to reduce and maintain their weight (Wadden, Crerand, & Brock, 2005).

DIETING

Overall, dieting seems to lead to short-term weight loss, although it has very limited long-term success regardless of whether diets are self-controlled or managed through a structured program. In fact, most people regain most or all of the weight they lost within five years (Weiss, Galuska, Khan, Gillespie, & Serdula, 2007), largely because people stop adhering to the plan. An analogy that comes to mind (given our psychology background) is the medical treatment of conditions such as bipolar disorder or depression, where people decide to stop taking medication because they feel better. This happens quite often, and as expected, patients experience a relapse. The same kind of thing happens as weight loss occurs. It may start with breaking the regimen as a treat for "being good," which then leads to skipping a day because the day is already shot from the earlier treat, and so begins the slippery slope down the hill of weight regain.

This actually happened to Oprah Winfrey, who had a notorious history of rapid weight loss and regain. She went on a very low calorie liquid diet and proudly disclosed her loss of 67 pounds, donning some new outfits on the covers of prestigious magazines. A couple years later, she had gained all the weight back, claiming she would never diet again. Kirstie Alley is also well known for her battles with weight. Oddly enough, she went on the Oprah Winfrey show in 2006 showing off her 75-pound weight loss from following Jenny Craig. The following year, she went off Jenny Craig and gained back everything plus another eight pounds. She now has her own TV show, and her own commercial diet plan. To make matters worse, re-losing weight after gaining it back tends to be quite difficult, and weight cycling (losing and gaining and losing and gaining) has been linked to increased all-cause mortality and other health problems (Arnold, Newman, Cushman, Ding, & Kritchevsky, 2010).

The cards seem slightly stacked against us when it comes to dieting. After dieting and restricting intake, people tend to become more sensitive to palatable foods, putting them in danger of losing dietary control when surrounded by tasty high-calorie foods (which seems nearly constant in our obesogenic world). Compounding the problem because our body tries to maintain homeostasis, our metabolic rate goes down when we starve ourselves, such that when we do lose control after dieting, it does more damage (i.e., more weight gain) than it did before the dieting started.

The more time that elapses after the completion of a diet program, the greater weight regain that occurs, and the rate of weight regain over time (even beyond five years) does not level off (Mann et al., 2007). Thus, in the long term, dieting does not seem to do the trick, but it may help you fit into a particular suit or dress for a formal event in a few weeks. Although some evidence exists that long-term weight loss can occur from various diets (Brown et al., 2009), these studies are few and far between, and the average weight loss viewed as significant or "successful" can still be quite low. (Is a one pound loss really a success?) One review of dieting studies that included 17 research publications from the 1930s through 1999 found only a 15% long-term success rate (Ayyad & Andersen, 2000). Here, the definition of success was either maintenance of 100% of initial weight loss (so losing only three pounds but maintaining it over time would be a "success") or maintenance of at least 9 to 11 kg of initial weight loss (about 20 pounds). With that said, there are what seem to be as many diets as there are stars in the night sky. We will try to review some common diets, as well as those that are kind of entertaining.

General Dieting Recommendations

As stated previously in the book, one of the major causes of obesity is an excess of calories consumed compared with energy used. Thus, one of the seemingly simple and logical ways to address obesity is to reduce the amount of calories consumed. General guidelines for diets (National Collaborating Centre for Primary Care, 2006) indicate that:

- Diets that lead to consuming 600 fewer calories per day than what is needed to stay the same weight, in combination with expert support and regular follow-up, are most often recommended for sustainable weight loss.
- Low-calorie diets (diets consisting of 1,000–1,600 calories/ day) are less likely to be nutritionally balanced.
- Very-low-calorie diets (less than 1,000 calories/day; other definitions include less than 800 calories/day) can be used for individuals who have reached a plateau in weight loss. The exact definition of these diets is somewhat arbitrary and varies; however, the general guideline is that very-low-calorie diets should be followed for, at most, 12 consecutive weeks,

or intermittently with a low-calorie diet while under medical supervision. The intent is rapid weight loss rather than a sustainable pattern of eating.

● Diets consisting of less than 600 calories/day should be used only under clinical supervision.

Even though these different diets lead to different degrees of weight loss in the short term, a direct comparison of different diets generally produces no significant differences in the long term (Brown et al., 2009), likely due to the common denominator that people tend to regain their weight. This goes for interventions that also include behavior therapy or exercise; the comparisons do not suggest that adding these components to diets lead to increased weight loss long-term. Why? Same answer—if you can't stick to the regimen and revert to old habits, weight loss will not be sustained.

As for the pediatric population, the evidence does not support any particular diet for children or adolescents at this time (Spear et al., 2007). This may be because children require energy and nutrients to grow properly. While some particular dietary programs have been found moderately effective, such as the Traffic Light Diet, they were also paired with various other components simultaneously (e.g., counseling, contracts, praise and modeling, self-monitoring training, exercise), making it difficult to determine the impact of the diet alone. An additional concern is that dieting in youth, either to lose weight or simply maintain weight, is associated with later risk of obesity even after controlling for baseline BMI (Neumark-Sztainer et al., 2006; Neumark-Sztainer, Wall, Haines, Story, & Eisenberg, 2007), indicating that this risk is not simply due to pre-existing overweight or obesity.

Mediterranean Diet

Anyone who has traveled to Europe, particularly the Mediterranean, will likely notice that the people seem generally thin (well, thinner than in the United States). This may be difficult to explain given that they eat lots of cheeses, oils, and other goodies that are often on our bad-to-eat list. How is this possible?

The Mediterranean diet has been examined in an attempt to explain the increased longevity and reduced mortality in certain regions compared with the United States. This diet is typically characterized by plant-based foods (nuts, legumes, fruits, seeds), fresh local ingredients, olive oil, a glass of wine with meals, regular consumption of fresh fish and seafood, moderate consumption of dairy, poultry and eggs, and low consumption of red meat (Buckland, Bach, & Serra-Majem, 2008). A review of 21 studies revealed that more than half found significant weight loss and reduction in obesity for those on the Mediterranean diet; the others saw no association between the diet and obesity (Buckland et al., 2008). Thus, the Mediterranean diet shows some promise, although the evidence is not overwhelming. Our personal research in Italy has found the diet to be delicious, though.

Low-Carbohydrate Diet

The low-carbohydrate diet, such as the Atkins diet (Dr. Atkins has sold more than 10 million copies of his book describing the diet), is vastly different from conventional diets. It consists of low-carb, high-fat, and high-protein consumption. Some studies have demonstrated short-term weight loss (e.g., 8%–10% after 8 weeks and 24 weeks, respectively; Foster et al., 2003). However, Foster et al. found that while initial weight loss (six months) was greater than that seen for a conventional diet, this difference was not significant after one year. Other studies have found no major differences between the long-term effects of the low-carbohydrate and conventional diets (Demol et al., 2009). This is likely because of difficulty in maintaining either diet for the long term, as is the problem for pretty much every diet.

Liquid Diets and Meal Replacements

Liquid diets often refer to the (very) low-calorie diets described above. These diets typically consist of drinking some kind of mixture of concentrated ingredients to ensure that certain nutritional needs are met with a minimal number of calories. These are considered safe provided that there is some level of medical monitoring, although some associated risks include gallstones, cold intolerance, hair loss, headache, fatigue, dizziness, muscle cramps, and constipation (Tsai & Wadden, 2006). Unsupervised liquid diets can lead to cardiac complications or even death.

Meal replacements consist of replacing meals with shakes or other prepackaged diet entrées. They have been found to be a useful adjunct to weight-loss interventions and lead to weight loss in the early stages of dieting. Comparisons of low-calorie diets and meal replacement strategies tend to yield similar degrees of weight loss or slightly greater weight loss with meal replacement (e.g., Heymsfield, van Mierlo, van der Knaap, Heo, & Frier, 2003; LeCheminant, Jacobsen, Hall, & Donnelly, 2005). Similar to other interventions, though, adherence to meal replacement strategies tends to wane after a time; after all, eating the same foods every day gets boring and is difficult to sustain. On a positive note, some research suggests that adherence to meal replacement diets may be higher than conventional weight-loss diets (Noakes, Foster, Keogh, & Clifton, 2004). In some respects, it is easier to adhere to a meal replacement diet because the decisions surrounding what foods to eat are made for you. Have a shake, end of story. No need to decipher nutrition information for the choices on your favorite take-out menu.

Caloric Restriction and Life Expectancy

Some research on rodents (and currently on primates) has found that caloric restriction while maintaining basic nutritional needs can lead to a host of positive effects, including reduced incidence of type 2 diabetes, atherosclerosis, obesity, dyslipidemia, even cancer; and accordingly, increased life span. At present, the effects of a lifetime of caloric restriction on the life span of humans are unknown, although it may lead to many of the same health benefits that are seen in rodents and primates, which are directly linked to life span (Fontana, 2009). More research is clearly needed before any serious claims are made. Regardless, maintaining a calorie restricted (typically about two thirds of your caloric requirements), yet nutritionally viable, diet for the long term has proven extremely difficult, and quite honestly, unreasonable for most people.

The Most Ridiculous, Absurd, and Over-Hyped Diets of 2010 (Koskie, 2010)

DietsinReview (2009) offered a sampling of diets that are sure to entertain. For example:

- Twinkie diet, which entails (surprise surprise) eating mostly Twinkies along with a variety of other cookies and packaged pastries (one third of the diet came from vegetables, a multivitamin, and a protein shake). This actually came from a Kansas State University nutrition professor named Mark Haub, who attempted to prove that total calories consumed (rather than where the calories come from) made the difference. He ate only 1,800 calories a day, but the calories came mostly from sugary, non-nutritious sources. Surprisingly, he lost 27 pounds over two months, body fat dropped by nine percentage points, his BMI dropped nearly four points, and his cholesterol and ratio of LDL to HDL improved. In the end, this of course is unsustainable and pretty ridiculous when it comes to overall health. Kids, don't try this at home.
- The Baby Food Diet, which entails eating those cute little jars of baby food. Like pureed peas and carrots? Not only is this pricey, but the amount of food offered in these servings is

intended for babies, not adults, and will leave you malnourished (and looking ridiculous in the break room at work).

● The Tapeworm Diet calls for people to swallow a tapeworm parasite that will assist in breaking down your digestive system, leaving you with less of an appetite. Sadly, it will also land you in the hospital and can possibly kill you. In case you were curious, tapeworms are not high in protein.

● The hCG Diet entails injecting a female pregnancy hormone combined with a 500-calorie per day diet. Yikes.

Popular Commercial Programs

Nutrisystem, Jenny Craig, and Weight Watchers are some of the more popular commercial programs available, although many exist. Interestingly, research has failed to show any major positive impacts for severely obese individuals. Unlike medications, the Federal Trade Commission (FTC) monitors advertising claims of the various commercial programs, although the programs are not required to submit any formal data for review; therefore, few data are available to review.

Weight Watchers has previously completed some randomized studies of the effectiveness of the program, one of which led to an average loss of 5% initial body weight after one year among those completing the program, and 3% weight loss at two-year follow-up (Heshka et al., 2003). A review from Tsai and Wadden (2005) noted that Weight Watchers was the only commercial program with data from scientifically sound studies supporting its use, albeit for a very modest weight loss. However, since that time a study from Foster et al. (2009) revealed the short-term efficacy of Nutrisystem (note that Nutrisystem funded the research).

Truth be told, many of the commercial programs utilize many of the same methods that include either low-calorie diets or meal replacements (or both) combined with some kind of behavior modification and physical activity. This is likely to lead to short-term weight loss, logically. Without knowing the long-term impact, however, it's somewhat premature to consider any of these programs "effective" in addressing obesity.

PHYSICAL ACTIVITY

We will keep this short and simple—both physical activity and exercise are very good for you (save dangerous sport-related injuries or overdoing it). Regular exercise can improve weight, lipid profiles, cholesterol, strength, blood pressure, and insulin resistance, and lets you feel more comfortable in a bathing suit. Increasing physical activity focuses on the other side of the energy equation, as many believe (especially for youth) that the increase in obesity is caused by sedentary lifestyles, video games, TV, and less time "scraping your knees on the pavement."

Unfortunately, much like diet programs, long-term weight loss from structured exercise programs is modest at best, in part due to the minimal adherence to these exercise programs over time. Let's face it—it's hard to keep up that 6:00 am hour-long spinning class, or the lap swimming during your lunch break. Without dietary changes, intense physical activity interventions produce weight losses of only about three to five pounds (Goldberg & King, 2007). This is not to say that maintaining a regimen of exercise throughout the life span will not lead to weight loss or prevent weight gain; but trying to adhere to structured exercise programs over the long haul is exceptionally difficult. The likelihood that those participants will continue on their own is small. Still, even short-term exercise programs do improve some other health indicators, even if the weight loss is not substantial. Further, interventions that target physical activity among children and adolescents do show more promise in reducing BMI (Spear et al., 2007).

BEHAVIOR (COGNITIVE-BEHAVIOR) AND LIFESTYLE MODIFICATION

Behavior modification strategies encompass an array of strategies that may attempt to address thought patterns (cognitive), behavior, or a combination (cognitive-behavioral). Cognitive-behavioral strategies, such as goal setting, stimulus control, and cognitive restructuring are used to help people adopt and maintain changes in their thoughts and related patterns of eating and physical activity (Wing, 2002). For example, cognitive-behavior programs may attempt to change a person's beliefs and attitudes surrounding food and weight, thereby translating to changes in behavior. We were watching one of our favorite shows one evening, Top Chef, and one of the contestants literally said, "Healthy food sucks. Unhealthy food tastes good." This is not an uncommon belief, but one that may actually be modified. Some possible cognitive or behavior modification strategies are listed in Table 5.1.

Reviews of randomized trials demonstrate that such interventions, typically delivered in 15 to 24 weekly group sessions, produce an average weight loss of approximately 5% to 10% of initial body weight (Perri & Corsica, 2002; Wadden et al., 2005; Wing, 2002). Such losses also lead to reductions in risk factors for heart disease and type 2 diabetes (Diabetes Prevention Program Research Group, 2002).

Interestingly, Internet-based behavior modification programs were found to result in weight loss, although to a slightly lesser degree than programs with in-person meetings (Harvey-Berino et al., 2010). Internet programs may be an alternative when barriers such as lack of program availability, transportation difficulties, and time constraints reduce compliance with more traditional in-person programs.

Unfortunately, much of the weight from these behavior modification programs is often regained at follow-up; like

TABLE 5.1 BEHAVIOR MODIFICATION STRATEGIES

Cognitive	Behavioral	Cognitive–Behavioral
Recognition and acceptance of weight stability as a goal	Eating a healthy diet (see Dieting section)	Goal setting
Identification and moderation of unrealistic expectations	Participation in an active lifestyle	Stimulus control (identifying triggers or barriers preventing weight loss and addressing them)
Problem solving to overcome obstacles to weight maintenance	Self-monitoring of food intake and weight	Cognitive restructuring
Addressing body image concerns	Offering incentives for meeting certain goals	
Reframing negative thoughts and attributions	Planning for the future by creating a personal weight maintenance plan	
Sustaining motivation		
Relapse-prevention training to overcome setbacks and actively cope with problems		

many other approaches, weight loss is rarely maintained once structured interventions and therapies end.

PRESCRIPTION MEDICATION

Very few FDA-approved prescription weight loss drugs have been made commercially available. These drugs are typically prescribed to individuals with a BMI over 30, or 27 if they have obesity-related medical issues. They are approved for short-term use (several weeks or months, not years), although orlistat can be used for up to two years (also commonly known as the OTC product Alli). The drugs on the market now work either by suppressing appetite (e.g., sibutramine, phentermine), or by blocking the absorption of fat (e.g., orlistat).

There are several other types of drugs that are prescribed "off-label," meaning that doctors will prescribe them for weight loss even though they are intended for some other purpose. For example, some antidepressant medications (e.g., Wellbutrin) and some antiseizure medications (e.g., Topamax) have been found to produce weight loss as a side effect. There are, of course, other side effects to consider when going this route.

In one recent study (Hendricks, Rothman, & Greenway, 2009), 98% of physicians surveyed reportedly used medication to treat patients with obesity, and most used phentermine on a long-term basis, despite its approval as a short-term medication only. Orlistat was prescribed for only 8% of patients treated medically for obesity.

Losses of 7% to 10% of initial body weight have been reported with six months of medical prescription medication treatment (typically orlistat or sibutramine), and these losses were reportedly maintained at two-year follow-up, provided patients continue to take the medication (James et al., 2000). However, once people stop taking the medication, they generally regain the weight, likely because people tend to maintain the same activity and dietary habits that contributed to obesity in the first place. Most significant weight loss associated with medical treatment is typically attributable to the co-occurrence of structured lifestyle changes (Aronne, Nelinson, & Lillo, 2009; Spear et al., 2007).

Side Effects of Medication

Several problems have cropped up over the past several years with weight-loss medications. A Saturday Night Live sketch actually poked fun at the potential problems that can come from using weight-loss medications, with a great deal of exaggeration for good measure. Jim Carrey hosted, and did a mock infomercial on a new weight-loss treatment that allowed him to lose 155 pounds in three and a half weeks. When an "audience member" asked whether it was unhealthy, Carrey's character twitched and said, "When I close my eyes, all I see are spiders and snails. My skin is clammy. My mouth is very dry. I think of suicide nonstop. And five minutes ago, I vomited the strangest colors into my stage manager's fanny pack. But you know what? The main side effect is, these days when I'm wearing a blue suit, and I yawn, people don't try to stuff a letter into my mouth!" Another endorsement of the fake product said (more like screamed), "By using your method, I really lost weight fast. Probably too fast. The stress you put on my body made me slip into the bowels of a red nightmare. I sleep in my oven. My hair falls out in clumps. I cry when I see a tree, and I burn symbols into my house pets with a curling iron. But it's worth it, because, these days, when I'm wearing a black jumpsuit, I look like a closed umbrella!" This is clearly an incredible exaggeration, but as the old adage says, there's a grain of truth in every joke.

One side effect of orlistat (which blocks the absorption of fat) is "liquid gas" (in other words, diarrhea—but apparently consumers don't like to hear diarrhea listed as a potential side effect in a commercial) as well as "oily spotting, loose stools, and more frequent stools that may be hard to control" (GlaxoSmithKline, 2011). Alli's Web site goes further to state that the undigested fat passes through your body, and while it is not harmful, "you may recognize it in the toilet as something that looks like the oil on top of a pizza" (GlaxoSmithKline, 2011). By the way, what's for dinner? We want to point out that when leaving the product's Web site and searching for other side effects, we found more potential side effects, including rectal discomfort, stomach pain, headaches, anxiety, irregular menstrual periods, nausea, loss of appetite, dark urine, yellowing of the skin or eyes, fatigue, rash, and difficulty swallowing (National

Center for Biotechnology Information, U.S. National Library of Medicine, 2010). More recently, a consumer rights advocacy group called Public Citizen called for a ban on orlistat due to increased risk of side effects, including liver damage, pancreatitis, and kidney stones (Salahi, 2011). Other side effects from some of the other appetite suppressant drugs can cause things such as headaches, sleeplessness, and increased heart rate.

More extreme side effects have been known to occur as well, including the potential for drug abuse and even death. For example, a drug used to treat obesity commonly known as Fen-Phen was pulled from the market after it was found to cause heart problems. Sibutramine (also called Meridia) was just pulled from markets in 2010 because of the increased risk of heart attacks and strokes. Several other drugs have recently been rejected by the FDA (e.g., Contrave, Qnexa, rimonabant, and lorcaserin) because there is insufficient evidence that they work, or the risk of negative side effects, including increased risk of heart problems or cancer, was too great compared with the small benefit that they offer. New drugs are constantly under development, as pharmaceutical companies seek to discover a magic bullet (and huge money maker).

OVER-THE-COUNTER

Orlistat (Alli) is now sold OTC, and is the only OTC medication that has actually been scientifically proven effective (because it was previously a prescription medication, it had to undergo safety and efficacy studies). As such, it's also the only OTC weight-loss drug that has FDA approval. There are hundreds or thousands of other OTC products claiming to help people to lose weight, with typically little to no evidence suggesting that they work, despite the gorgeous model posing on the label. Many pills contain caffeine, which is essentially just a diuretic, so you may lose weight, but it's just water weight. There is also no evidence to suggest that they are safe, and in some cases, they may be harmful.

Medications sold OTC do not have to undergo the same rigorous testing and safety measures of prescription medications. Because there are so many OTC drugs, the FDA only reviews the active ingredients commonly found in OTC products and approves use of those ingredients rather than the OTC products themselves; thus, OTC medications do not need preapproval and can be sold without any individual testing. The FDA does make some surprise inspections of drug manufacturers, but there just aren't enough hours in the day to get to all of them. In contrast, the FDA has to thoroughly test and pre-approve prescription medications (which is partly why they cost so much).

Now, if a new product came out called LoseWeight, and then you lost an eyeball one week after trying it, you could call the FDA to investigate. Depending on the severity of the issue (e.g., 50 people made similar calls, which have been tied directly to the product), the FDA can request modifications from the manufacturer, help improve instructions or warning labels, request name changes, or work with the manufacturer to issue a recall, but the response is reactive rather than preventive, and the FDA cannot actually *enforce* a recall. As of the writing of this book, the Drug Safety and Accountability Act has been introduced to Congress, but has yet to be passed. This bill calls for increased FDA authority over the production, safety, and recall of drugs sold in the United States, including OTC drugs. Stay tuned.

Herbal

There are thousands of herbal diet pills available. Like OTC medication, herbal remedies do not have to be evaluated by the FDA to be sold. As such, there are some concerns with the lack of rigorous scientific study of supplements on the market and their effectiveness in helping people to lose weight (hopefully you will agree that the highly photo-shopped "before" and "after" images endorsed by some actor in a white lab coat do not qualify as evidence). Unfortunately, many people incorrectly assume that all herbal medications are natural and safe.

One particular analysis (Hasani-Ranjbar, Nayebi, Larijani, & Abdollahi, 2009) reviewed 77 studies examining the effects of herbal medications on weight loss and obesity (58 animal studies and 19 human studies, 11 of which were double-blind randomized controlled trials). Human studies generally revealed loss of body weight, body fat, decreases in waist and hip circumference, decreases in appetite and food intake, and few significant adverse effects associated with herbal obesity treatments. The most adverse effects were seen for herbal medications containing ephedra and caffeine. Authors note, however, that several clinical trials would lose patients to negative side effects, and other clinical trials were never completed (and thus not included in this review), as they had to discontinue the trial after discovering certain negative reactions to the supplements. The criterion for "success" in this review was if the study showed a "statistically significant" difference in weight loss between the group taking the herbal medication and those taking placebo (or in two studies, from pretreatment to post-treatment). This could mean that the treatment group lost two pounds, while the placebo group stayed the same. The review did not specify the overall magnitude of weight losses seen in studies of herbal remedies. In addition, this review did acknowledge the need to assess long-term impacts.

On the contrary to this review, there is evidence that some pills and supplements can actually be dangerous. Because supplements are barely regulated, they may contain elements that have some nasty side effects, and it can take years to discover that these "natural remedies" are in fact harmful. As noted by Chan (2009), some antiobesity herbal products may contain highly toxic herbs or herbal laxatives, and these disclosures may not be present on the label. There have been several instances where the FDA had to ban the sale of pills containing certain ingredients, such as Ephedra (which is like a natural form of amphetamines). As a result, Chan concludes that "herbal antiobesity products are not recommended as part of a weight-loss program, since they have unpredictable amounts of active ingredients, and unpredictable and potentially harmful effects." (p. 455). Other studies mirror this message (e.g., Senturk, Ozdabakoglu, & Baran, 2008). More recently, a group of researchers in Germany found that an array of herbal weight-loss supplements that claim to lead to weight loss did not lead to any significant weight loss compared with a placebo pill (International Association for the Study of Obesity, 2010).

In sum, some herbal remedies are potentially helpful, although likely yield no significant long-term weight loss and some are potentially dangerous. Until there can be more oversight over the production and commercial sales of such products, you will be hard pressed to find a full endorsement of herbal weight-loss products from the scientific community.

Medication Use with Children and Adolescents

Few guidelines are available when it comes to the use of medication for obesity treatment among children and adolescents (Spear et al., 2007). At present, only orlistat has been FDA approved for obesity treatment among the pediatric population (sibutramine was as well, although as stated above, it has since been pulled from the shelves). The general thinking is that weight loss medication should be reserved for youth with extreme obesity and who have had minimal success with other alternatives (e.g., diet or exercise programs, lifestyle modification). In addition, as is the case for adults, medical management should be paired with lifestyle management techniques, particularly to help youth maintain weight loss after discontinuing medication (Spear et al., 2007).

SURGERY

Over 200,000 individuals undergo weight-loss surgery in the United States each year. Weight-loss surgery tends to be reserved for individuals with severe obesity and other comorbid health conditions who have also had little to no success with previous attempts at weight loss. The general guideline is that weight-loss surgery should be a last resort intervention for adults, and only appropriate when the following conditions have been met:

- BMI over 40, or 35 with comorbidities (e.g., diabetes or hypertension).
- Other methods have not resulted in significant and sustainable weight loss after six months.
- The person commits to long-term follow-up, as lifelong medical monitoring is necessary (NHLBI, 2000).
- The person receives intensive medical management.
- The person is fit for anesthesia and surgery.
- The person has received a psychological evaluation to determine if any factors may interfere with the success of the surgery (e.g., eating disorders, mental disorders interfering with postoperative care, depression) and if psychological or psychiatric treatment is needed as an initial step.
- If BMI is over 50, surgery may be considered as a first option.

Surgery, generally speaking, is a highly effective method resulting in significant and sustained weight loss for more than five years in the majority of patients (NHLBI, 2000), and in one cohort study after 10 years (Sjostrom et al., 2004). In fact, a systematic review of 26 research studies (Picot et al., 2009) revealed that bariatric surgery (weight-loss surgery) was generally more effective than other weight-loss options. Other positive effects included short-term improved quality of life for some, as well as a reduction in comorbidities. Surgery has been said to be the only "cure" for type 2 diabetes (Coleman & Phillips, 2010).

Bariatric surgery is generally not recommended for children or adolescents. That said, a panel of surgeons recommended that if pediatric patients are to undergo surgery, they should be physically mature, have a BMI between 40 and 50 with significant comorbidities, and meet the other characteristics noted above for adults (Inge et al., 2004). Further, a general recommendation is that girls be at least 13 years of age and boys 15 years of age prior to even considering bariatric surgery. However, each individual case should be considered separately rather than following a rigid guideline.

Several methods of bariatric surgery are available and can be divided into categories of restricting intake, reducing absorption of food, and a combination (both restricting intake and reducing absorption of energy by the body). Below are four commonly used surgical techniques, although others, including the intragastric balloon and implantable gastric stimulation, may become more prevalent in the future.

Gastric Bypass

Normally, when we eat food, it passes through the stomach to the small intestines. This is where most of the nutrients and calories are absorbed by the body. What's left passes through the large intestine, and then, our body disposes of it. Gastric bypass modifies this digestive process by making the stomach smaller (restricting intake) and re-routing some of the internal wiring to bypass part of the small intestines (reducing absorption by the body; see Figure 5.1). Therefore, gastric bypass is considered a combination surgical therapy. The Roux-en-Y gastric bypass (stomach stapling) is the most common form of gastric bypass. Put simply, the stomach is sectioned off using staples or a plastic band, creating a small pouch at the top of the stomach. This smaller pouch (the new stomach) is connected to the middle of the small intestine, which therefore bypasses the remainder of the stomach and a large part of the small intestines. Less is absorbed, and because the stomach is so much smaller, fullness and satiety occur with small amounts of food.

Gastric bypass is highly effective, and in fact generally more effective than the other procedures listed below (Picot et al., 2009). However, this procedure (like any other surgery) comes with some potential side effects, including hernia, staples

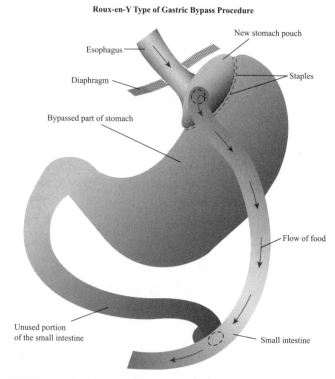

Roux-en-Y Type of Gastric Bypass Procedure

New stomach pouch

Esophagus

Staples

Diaphragm

Bypassed part of stomach

Flow of food

Unused portion
of the small intestine

Small intestine

FIGURE 5.1 A depiction of Roux-en-Y gastric bypass surgery.

pulling loose, ulcers, nausea after eating, iron and vitamin B12 deficiencies, anemia, osteoporosis, leaks at the stomach and small intestine connection, and other complications associated with surgery.

Laparoscopic Adjustable Gastric Banding (a.k.a. Lap Band)

This is considered the least invasive[1] bariatric surgery option (Picot et al., 2009). A constricting ring is placed around the top of the stomach. Essentially, this is similar to gastric bypass, although it does not reroute the small intestines and instead simply makes the stomach smaller. Currently, the bands come with an inflatable balloon in the lining that allows for adjustment of the size of the modified stomach pouch. Gastric banding is also a reversible procedure. Potential side effects include injury to the spleen or esophagus, wound infection, band slippage or migration, a leak in the new stomach pouch, nausea, and acid reflux. Perhaps another side effect that may be particularly frustrating is the need for significant adjustments or removal of the band as some have suggested that the band fails upward of 30% of the time (Picot et al., 2009).

Use of the lap-band procedure among adolescents has increased substantially in recent years. In fact, one study found that use of the lap band increased nearly sevenfold from 2005 to 2007, whereas gastric bypass among adolescents slightly decreased (Jen et al., 2010). The lap-band procedure may become even more popular in coming years, as the FDA is considering approval of this device for use in obese individuals with a BMI of 35 or 30 in the presence of comorbidities.

Biliopancreatic Diversion (With Duodenal Switch)

This procedure, which has been modified from the original biliopancreatic division, entails actual removal of a part of the stomach to limit intake, although the remaining pouch is larger than the pouches usually used with gastric bypass or the lap band. Similar to the gastric bypass, the small intestine is rearranged, although this is done so in a different way. This procedure separates the channel of food in the small intestine from the channel of digestive juices, such that they only meet at the "end" of the small intestine, leading to reduced absorption of food. This means that a lot of food goes through your system undigested (and not absorbed as calories).

Some side effects may include loose stools, ulcers, offensive body odors, loss of energy, hair loss, protein malnutrition, chronic diarrhea, excess gas, osteoporosis, night blindness (due to malabsorption of vitamin A), or leakages near the stitching.

Sleeve Gastrectomy

This procedure leads to the stomach being reduced in size vertically to about 25%, ensuring that stomach function and digestion remain unaltered by leaving the pyloric valve intact. This procedure is irreversible. In some cases, this procedure is enough to lead to clinically significant weight loss. Many times, a gastric bypass or a duodenal switch may be added. A sleeve gastrectomy is often used as a first step when one is determined to be at high risk from bariatric surgery (Picot et al., 2009). This is a relatively minor surgery with fewer risks and potential side effects than gastric bypass or duodenal switch, in part because it does not impact digestion. However, potential complications include nausea from overeating and other postoperative complications.

OTHER POPULAR TRENDS

Active Video Gaming

Active video gaming (if you've been living under a rock) describes those great new video games that actually require body movement to play rather than simply pressing some buttons. This smartly ties the growing trend of children playing video games to the need for increased activity levels. To no surprise, active video gaming increases energy expenditure, and is safe, fun, and engaging. One study found that active video gaming is actually comparable to moderate-intensity walking (Graf, Pratt, Hester, & Short, 2009). To be sure, in order to enjoy the physical benefits of active video gaming, those playing must—well—be active. Sitting on the couch and shifting your wrist to hit a digital tennis ball will not do much for your weight or health.

Financial Incentives

A meta-analysis revealed that financial incentives, such as paying study participants for adherence to exercise or diet plans, weight loss, or attendance at sessions, do not have a significant effect on weight loss after 1 year and after 18 months (Paul-Ebhohimhen & Avenell, 2008). This seems somewhat consistent with our general understanding of behavior modification insomuch as reward presented immediately (food, enjoyment) are more salient than delayed rewards (e.g., money after a weigh-in each week).

Biggest Loser Competitions

The popularity of the reality TV show Biggest Loser, where people achieve transformational weight losses, has created somewhat of a mass movement to turn weight loss into a competitive sport. In fact, we have seen various groups of coworkers or faculty in school buildings begin a Biggest Loser competition with weekly weigh-ins. Some schools have even suggested this for the students.

Biggest Loser is an entertaining TV show, and the results of the contestants speak for themselves. What people do not realize is that much more goes into that weight loss than a few workout montages, good looking personal trainers, brightly colored matching t-shirts, and some creative elimination challenges. If you have quick enough reflexes to pause the show at the end, you will see some disclaimers, including the availability of medical staff at all times, the rigorous training involved, and the warnings to not jump into similar attempts at weight loss without consulting a professional. This is in part because of the risks associated with rapid weight loss (see liquid diets above).

Some other issues related to Biggest Loser are the same issues associated with almost every single intervention discussed in this chapter; long-term weight loss is questionable, as the intensive diet and exercise regimen is nearly impossible to sustain. It rewards quick, short-term loss, which most of the time leads to regain soon afterwards. These competitions tend to reward weight loss, instead of healthy behaviors or lifestyle changes. This would mean that the nutrition professor who ate mostly Twinkies could have won. Competitions can be motivating and fun, but they should focus on healthy behaviors, such as intake of vegetables or steps recorded on a pedometer.

Clinical Hypnosis

Clinical hypnosis, or hypnotherapy (i.e., not "stage hypnosis" or the "watch the watch" stuff used for entertainment purposes), is commonly attempted for weight loss, although the available research has not been able to conclusively support or refute any claims of effectiveness (Najm & Lie, 2010). Some have suggested that it may improve compliance with the treatment program over the long-term, which as we note throughout, is a major barrier to weight loss. However, the jury is out.

Acupuncture

Some have suggested that acupuncture may support efforts at weight loss. One recent study applied an intervention to two groups of obese individuals, where one group received a dietician's advice, while the other group also received acupuncture and psychotherapy (Buevich, Bozhko, Larisa, & Fedorov, 2010). The acupuncture and psychotherapy group had more positive results for weight loss, which the authors partly attributed to acupuncture reducing appetite, increasing metabolism, and improving internal organ function. However, as noted by Najm and Lie (2010), most studies of acupuncture (including Buevich et al., 2010) are of short duration and are poorly controlled (you can imagine it is hard to "blind" participants to whether they are in acupuncture treatment group or not). Preliminary evidence may support its use on a short-term basis in conjunction with other treatments, but more research is needed.

Colonics

For those don't know, colonics flushes out the colon by infusing water into the rectum and removing waste through a tube. Colon hydrotherapists claim that the procedure can lead to weight loss, although the basis of many of these claims are largely unfounded (Seow-Choen, 2009), not to mention, extremely unpleasant sounding.

Other Fads

The list is long, as new diet plans come out all the time. Table 5.2 shows just some of the most popular diets of 2009

TABLE 5.2 POPULAR DIETS IN 2009

Acai diet	Many health benefits from the acai berry, although not likely to lead to any substantial weight loss.
Hydroxycut	Claims to lead to weight loss and increase energy. Meanwhile, the FDA tried to put a recall on the product due to liver damage.
Slim shots	A creamer for coffees or beverages that allegedly activates the hunger center in the brain to control appetite.
South Beach diet	One of the more popular low-carb diets that now incorporates more exercise and strength training.
Apple cider vinegar diet	Considered a detox cleanse. Detox cleanses typically aim to remove toxins and poisons from the body, and usually include a strict diet and reduction in calories consumed.
Lemonade diet	Another detox diet that consists of consuming lemon juice, maple syrup, cayenne pepper, and water for 45 days. Yum.
Cabbage soup diet	Pretty simple. Eat lots of cabbage soup and veggies and consume very few calories throughout the day.

(DietsinReview, 2009). Reviewing the merits of each plan is beyond the purview of this book, but suffice it to say none is likely to be a panacea for the obesity epidemic.

CONTROVERSIES IN TREATMENT

Here are just a few of the issues and controversies being discussed in the world of obesity treatment.

Liposuction

Liposuction entails the removal of fat below the skin. Seems great, right? Got some extra fat—no problem, just vacuum it out. The procedure is often incorrectly perceived as a quick and easy weight loss fix for obese individuals. However, it could take numerous liposuction treatments to notice any significant weight loss, causing significant trauma to the body. With that said, some studies have demonstrated improvements in various obesity-related risk factors (cardiovascular risk factors, insulin resistance) following liposuction, though many other studies have not shown these effects (Klein et al., 2004). Therefore, some controversy exists regarding its use for weight loss. Regardless, as Berry and Davies (2010) note, "Liposuction is not a panacea for obesity, and patients are not always cognizant of this."

TOFI—Weight and Weight Loss Is Not the Only Indicator for Health

TOFI is not a meat-substitute, but a relatively new and uncommon term that stands for "Thin on the Outside, Fat on the Inside," and describes individuals who maintain a normal weight although carry a great deal of fat stored around vital organs (e.g., heart, liver, pancreas) and muscles. This can be true of individuals who are not overweight or obese by BMI standards, but still maintain high levels of internal fat. Importantly, it presents the same risks to health as excess weight. The take-home message is that weight, BMI, and even waist circumference are not the only indicators of fat in the body and related health. This is a fairly new concept, however, so there is not a ton of available information addressing the issue of internal fat in the obesity literature. We suspect there will be more to come on this in the future.

Long-Term Results (Stink)

A reduction of 5% to 10% of body weight can have significant benefits; however, if the lost weight is regained, those benefits may be reversed (Klein, 2001). Unfortunately, we have made it clear (we hope) that weight regain following the discontinuation of treatment is more the norm than the exception. A telephone survey of U.S. adults reported that whereas 21% of overweight or obese individuals who had lost weight successfully maintained a 10% weight loss at one year, only 11% maintained this loss for five years or more (McGuire, Wing, & Hill, 1999). Further, a meta-analysis of long-term weight-loss studies in the United States revealed that the overall reduction in body weight at 4.5-year follow-up was only 2.1% (Anderson, Konz, Frederich, & Wood, 2001). So for a person weighing 200 pounds to start, they manage to hold steady at 196 pounds nearly five years later. Not exactly impressive. As stated earlier in the chapter, the trends of weight regain do not seem to level off at five years, so many assume that maintenance of weight loss will likely continue to drop off as time passes.

One possible reason for this trend is the high "cost" (behavioral, financial, mental) of maintaining strict control of weight over time compared with the diminishing benefits of weight loss (Perri & Corsica, 2002). After all, losing weight and keeping it off requires a lot of work. Most people decide it is not worth it to put in the same level of effort when they no longer get the reward of pounds dropping off. Who wants to work that hard to just stay the same? Say someone wants to run a marathon. Training comes at a cost—financial (buying running shoes and gear), emotional (dealing with frustration, potential injury, turning down other fun activities to stay in shape), and mental (mental effort, pushing oneself); however, as progress continues towards the goal, the benefits of the training are obvious, and the costs pay off. The race eventually comes. Goal achieved. Post-race, maintaining this level of training seems to have diminished benefits. Without another race on the horizon, the "costs" become more obvious and salient compared with the "benefits" of continued training. Efforts drop off and soon it becomes difficult to run even a few miles. This alone becomes frustrating, causing the person to not want to run anymore. This frequently happens when individuals don't meet their expectations for weight loss, leading to feelings of hopelessness and personal failure, which in turn leads to abandoning the weight-loss efforts.

In contrast, the longer a person maintains an initial weight loss, the greater likelihood they will successfully maintain weight loss several years down the line. Further, those who do manage to maintain weight loss report using fewer strategies and less effort to do so as time goes on, suggesting that weight maintenance gets easier over time (Klem, Wing, Lang, McGuire, & Hill, 2000). In sum, only a small minority of people can truly maintain the lifestyle changes necessary to keep their weights down over the long haul.

Various other factors have been suggested as contributing to the success of long-term weight loss, including the amount of initial weight lost, length of interventions and continued professional support, activity level, control of overeating, self-monitoring of behaviors, internal motivation to lose weight, autonomy, psychological strength, stability, skills such as problem solving and coping, and level of social support (Elfhag &

Rossner, 2005). Risk of weight gain may increase with weight cycling, disinhibited eating, emotional eating, and having a passive reaction to problems (Elfhag & Rossner, 2005).

Unfortunately, maintaining a diet and self-control require a great deal of cognitive energy, making it nearly impossible to sustain this effort long term (Cohen & Farley, 2008). The more effort devoted to restraining our food cravings, the less cognitive reserves we have to devote to other tasks. Conversely, if we use up our mental reserves at work or school, we have less capacity to resist temptation in the candy store. One clever research study illustrated this by asking one group to refrain from eating cookies while completing a difficult puzzle, whereas the other group had to complete the same puzzle but could eat the cookies. The group eating the cookies completed the puzzle and sustained attention for 19 minutes, whereas the other group refraining from eating had to quit the puzzle after 8 minutes and reported feeling more tired (Baumeister, Bratslavsky, Muraven, & Tice, 1998). It seems that asking them to resist eating the cookies exhausted their cognitive reserves. Applied to weight-loss efforts, this means that the effort it takes to keep up with a weight-loss maintenance regimen means our brains are less able to deal with other problems (and vice versa).

Offering Surgical Options for Less Obese People

As noted earlier, bariatric surgery is typically reserved for severely obese individuals (40 BMI or higher; 35 with comorbidities). In December, 2010, an FDA advisory panel endorsed expanding use of the lap-band surgery to less obese individuals based on supportive research (BMI of 35 kg/m^2 or greater, or 30 kg/m^2 with comorbidities). This may lead not only to more people receiving coverage for such surgeries but also to the possibility that other surgical procedures for obesity may be approved for a wider audience in the future. Some have suggested that it will enable poor lifestyle choices because individuals now have the option for a quick fix. Others have projected that this may lead to increases in health care costs as our health insurance premiums go up to cover the likelihood of surgery for millions of people. Other opponents have said that opening up the possibility of surgery to so many people may result in an over-reliance on surgery over other less invasive (and less risky, and less expensive) strategies to reduce obesity. However, given the poor long-term outcomes of other strategies for weight loss, combined with the toll that obesity-related conditions and comorbidities take, perhaps making surgery more widely available is not such a bad thing.

SUMMARY

The outlook on most weight loss treatments is generally pretty poor, which may not be particularly surprising, given the steadily increasing prevalence of obesity. Various methods of treatment have been implemented, studied, and reviewed, and thousands more have been promoted or sold on the market without any oversight whatsoever. Although many options are available and potentially effective for short-term weight loss, few options have been found useful for significant and sustainable long-term loss. Surgery is generally very effective although it comes with a number of risks and is limited to a select population of individuals, leaving millions of overweight and obese people with few effective long-term treatment options. Given the continued rise in obesity prevalence in the United States and abroad, we anticipate new products and treatment methods to be developed, although new treatments should be considered with caution until long-term effectiveness and safety can be established.

NOTE

[1]Laparoscopic refers to a less invasive procedure where operations are completed through the use of very small incisions. Surgeons often use a laparoscope, which magnifies the images on a monitor, as opposed to opening up the entire abdomen.

REFERENCES

Anderson, J. W., Konz, E. C., Frederich, R. C., & Wood, C. L. (2001). Long-term weight-loss maintenance: A meta-analysis of US studies. *American Journal of Clinical Nutrition, 74,* 579–584.

Andreyeva, T., Long, M. W., Henderson, K. E., & Grode, G. M. (2010). Trying to lose weight: Diet strategies among Americans with overweight or obesity in 1996 and 2003. *Journal of the American Dietetic Association, 110*(4), 535–542.

Arnold, A. M., Newman, A. B., Cushman, M., Ding, J., & Kritchevsky, S. (2010). Body weight dynamics and their association with physical function and mortality in older adults: The Cardiovascular Health Study. *The Journals of Gerontology. Series A, Biological Sciences and Medical Sciences, 65,* 63–70.

Aronne, L. J., Nelinson, D. S., & Lillo, J. L. (2009). Obesity as a disease state: A new paradigm for diagnosis and treatment. *Clinical Cornerstone, 9,* 9–29.

Ayyad, C., & Andersen, T. (2000). Long-term efficacy of dietary treatment of obesity: A systematic review of studies published between 1931 and 1999. *Obesity Reviews, 1,* 113–119.

Baradel, L. A., Gillespie, C., Kicklighter, J. R., Doucette, M. M., Penumetcha, M., & Blanck, H. M. (2009). Temporal changes in trying to lose weight and recommended weight-loss strategies among overweight and obese Americans, 1996–2003. *Preventive Medicine, 49,* 158–164.

Baumeister, R. F., Bratslavsky, E., Muraven, M., & Tice, D. M. (1998). Ego depletion: Is the active self a limited resource? *Journal of Personality and Social Psychology, 74,* 1252–1265.

Benson, L., Baer, H. J., & Kaelber, D. C. (2009). Trends in the diagnosis of overweight and obesity in children and adolescents: 1999–2007. *Pediatrics, 123*, 153–158.

Berry, M. G., & Davies, D. (2010). Liposuction: A review of principles and techniques. *Journal of Plastic, Reconstructive & Aesthetic Surgery*, doi:10.1016/j.pjps.2010.11.018.

Brown, T., Avenell, A., Edmunds, L. D., Moore, H., Whittaker, V., Avery, L., & Summerbell, C. (2009). Systematic review of long-term lifestyle interventions to prevent weight gain and morbidity in adults. *Obesity Reviews, 10*, 627–638.

Buckland, G., Bach, A., & Serra-Majem, L. (2008). Obesity and the Mediterranean diet: A systematic review of observational and intervention studies. *Obesity Reviews, 9*, 582–593.

Buevich, V., Bozhko, A., Larisa, V., & Fedorov, A. (2010). Acupuncture and psychotherapy in the complex treatment of obesity. *Medical Acupuncture, 22*, 187–190.

Chan, T. Y. K. (2009). Potential risks associated with the use of herbal anti-obesity products. *Drug Safety, 32*, 453–456.

Cohen, D. A., & Farley, T. A. (2008). Eating as an automatic behavior. *Preventing Chronic Disease, 5*, 1–7.

Coleman, J., & Phillips, S. (2010). Bariatric surgery: A cutting-edge cure for type 2 diabetes? *New Zealand Medical Journal, 123*(1311), 65–68.

Demol, S., Yackobovitch-Gavan, M., Shalitin, S., Nagelberg, N., Gillon-Keren, M., & Phillip, M. (2009). Low-carbohydrate (low & high-fat) versus high-carbohydrate low-fat diets in the treatment of obesity in adolescents. *Acta Paediatrica, 98*, 346–351.

Diabetes Prevention Program Research Group. (2002). Reduction in the incidence of type 2 diabetes with lifestyle intervention or metformin. *New England Journal of Medicine, 346*, 393–403.

DietsinReview. (2009). *25 most popular diets of 2009.* Retrieved January 7, 2011, from http://www.dietsinreview.com/slideshows/25-most-popular-diets-of-2009/weight-watchers/

Dorsey, K. B., Wells, C., Krumholz, H. M., & Concato, J. C. (2005). Diagnosis, evaluation, and treatment of childhood obesity in pediatric practice. *Archives of Pediatrics & Adolescent Medicine, 159*, 632–638.

Dorsey, R. R., Eberhardt, M. S., & Ogden, C. L. (2009). Racial/ethnic differences in weight perception. *Obesity, 17*(4), 790–795.

Elfhag, K., & Rossner, S. (2005). Who success in maintaining weight loss? A conceptual review of factors associated with weight loss maintenance and weight regain. *Obesity Reviews, 6*, 67–85.

Fontana, L. (2009). The scientific basis of caloric restriction leading to longer life. *Current Opinion in Gastroenterology, 25*, 144–150.

Foster, G. D., Borradaile, K. E., Vander Veur, S. S., Shantz, K. L., Dilks, R. J., Goldbacher, E. M.,…Satz, W. (2009). The effects of a commercially available weight loss program among obese patients with type 2 diabetes: A randomized study. *Postgraduate Medicine, 121*, 113–118.

Foster, G. D., Wyatt, H. R., Hill, J. O., McGuckin, B. G., Brill, C., Mohammed, M. D.,…Klein, S. (2003). A randomized trial of a low-carbohydrate diet for obesity. *The New England Journal of Medicine, 348*, 2082–2090.

GlaxoSmithKline. (2011). *Alli faqs.* Retrieved January 11, 2011, from http://www.myalli.com/faq.aspx

Goldberg, J. H., & King, A. C. (2007). Physical activity and weight management across the lifespan. *Annual Review of Public Health, 28*, 145–170.

Graf, D. L., Pratt, L. V., Hester, C. N., & Short, K. R. (2009). Playing active video games increases energy expenditure in children. *Pediatrics, 124*, 534–540.

Harvey-Berino, J., West, D., Krukowski, R., Prewitt, E., VanBiervliet, A., Ashikaga, T., & Skelly, J. (2010). Internet delivered behavioral obesity treatment. *Preventive Medicine, 51*, 123–128.

Hasani-Ranjbar, S., Nayebi, N., Larijani, B., & Abdollahi, M. (2009). A systematic review of the efficacy and safety of herbal medicines used in the treatment of obesity. *World Journal of Gastroenterology, 15*, 3073–3085.

Hendricks, E. J., Rothman, R. B., & Greenway, F. L. (2009). How physician obesity specialists use drugs to treat obesity. *Obesity, 17*, 1730–1735.

Heshka, S., Anderson, J. W., Atkinson, R. L., Greenway, F. L., Hill, J. O., Phinney, S. D.,…Pi-Sunyer, F. X. (2003). Weight loss with self-help compared with a structured commercial program: A randomized trial. *Journal of the American Medical Association, 289*, 1792–1798.

Heymsfield, S. B., van Mierlo, C. A. J., van der Knaap, H. C. M., Heo, M., & Frier, H. I. (2003). Weight management using a meal replacement strategy: Meta and pooling analysis from six studies. *International Journal of Obesity, 27,* 537–549.

Huang, J. S., Becerra, K., Oda, T., Walker, E., Xu, R., Donohue, M.,...Breslow, A. (2007). Parental ability to discriminate the weight status of children: Results of a survey. *Pediatrics, 120,* 112–119.

Inge, T. H., Krebs, N. F., Garcia, V. F., Skelton, J. A., Guice, K. S., & Strauss, R. S. (2004). Bariatric surgery for severely overweight adolescents: Concerns and recommendations. *Pediatrics, 114,* 217–223.

International Association for the Study of Obesity. (2010, July). No evidence that popular slimming supplements facilitate weight loss, new research finds. *ScienceDaily.* Retrieved January 8, 2011, from http://www.sciencedaily.com/releases/2010/07/100712103445.htm

James, W. P., Astrup, A., Finer, N., Hilsted, J., Kopelman, P., Rossner, S.,...Van Gaal L. F. (2000). Effect of sibutramine on weight maintenance after weight loss: A randomized trial. STORM study group. Sibutramine trial of obesity reduction and maintenance. *Lancet, 356,* 2119–2125.

Johnson-Taylor, W. L., Fisher, R. A., Hubbard, V. S., Starke-Reed, P., & Eggers, P. S. (2008). The change in weight perception of weight status among the overweight: Comparison of NHANES III (1988–1994) and 1999–2004 NHANES. *International Journal of Behavioral Nutrition and Physical Activity, 5,* 9.

Jen, H. C., Rickard, D. G., Shew, S. B., Maggard, M. A., Slusser, W. M, Dutson, E. P., & DeUgarte, D. A. (2010). Trends and outcomes of adolescent bariatric surgery in California, 2005–2007. *Pediatrics, 126,* 746–753.

Klein, S. (2001). Outcome success in obesity. *Obesity Research, 9,* 354S–358S.

Klein, S., Fontana, L., Young, V. L., Coggan, A. R., Kilo, C., Patterson, B. W., & Mohammed, B. S. (2004). Absence of an effect of liposuction on insulin action and risk factors for coronary heart disease. *New England Journal of Medicine, 350,* 2549–2557.

Klem, M. L., Wing, R. R., Lang, W., McGuire, M. T., & Hill, J. O. (2000). Does weight loss maintenance become easier over time? *Obesity Research, 8,* 438–444.

Koskie, B. (2010). *The most ridiculous, absurd and over-hyped diets of 2010.* Retrieved December 17, 2010, from http://shine.yahoo.com/channel/health/the-most-ridiculous-absurd-and-over-hyped-diets-of-2010–2423016/

LeCheminant, J. D., Jacobsen, D. J., Hall, M. A., & Donnelly, J. E. (2005). A comparison of meal replacements and medication in weight maintenance after weight loss. *Journal of the American College of Nutrition, 24,* 347–353.

Lemon, S. C., Rosal, M. C., Zapka, J., Borg, A., & Andersen, V. (2009). Contributions of weight perceptions to weight loss attempts: Differences by body mass index and gender. *Body Image, 6*(2), 90–96.

Louthan, M. V., Lafferty-Oza, M. J., Smith, E. R., Hornang, C. A., Franco, S., & Theriot, J. A. (2005). Diagnosis and treatment frequency of overweight children and adolescents at well child visits. *Clinical Pediatrics, 44,* 57–61.

Mann, T., Tomiyama, A. J., Westling, E., Lew, A. M., Samuels, B., & Chatman, J. (2007). Medicare's search for effective obesity treatments. *American Psychologist, 62,* 220–233.

Marketdata Enterprises, Inc. (2009). *The U.S. Weight Loss and Diet Control Market.* Tampa, FL.

McGuire, M. T., Wing, R. R., Klem, M. L., & Hill, J. O. (1999). The behavioral characteristics of individuals who lose weight unintentionally. *Obesity Research, 7,* 485–490.

Najm, W., & Lie, D. (2010). Herbals used for diabetes, obesity, and metabolic syndrome. *Primary Care: Clinics in Office Practice, 37,* 237–254.

National Center for Biotechnology Information, U.S. National Library of Medicine. (2010). *Orlistat.* Retrieved December 17, 2010, from http://www.ncbi.nlm.nih.gov/pubmedhealth/PMH0000175

National Collaborating Centre for Primary Care. (2006). *Obesity: The prevention, identification, assessment and management of overweight and obesity in adults and children.* Retrieved December 7, 2010, from http://www.guideline.gov/content.aspx?id=10263

National Heart, Lung, and Blood Institute Obesity Education Initiative. (2000). *The Practical Guide: Identification, Evaluation, and Treatment of Overweight and Obesity in Adults.* Retrieved December 27, 2010, from http://www.nhlbi.nih.gov/guidelines/obesity/prctgd_c.pdf

Neumark-Sztainer, D., Wall, M., Guo, J., Story, M., Haines, J., & Eisenberg, M. E. (2006). Obesity, disordered eating, and eating disorders in a longitudinal study of adolescents: How do dieters fare 5 years later? *Journal of the American Dietetic Association, 106,* 559–568.

Neumark-Sztainer, D., Wall, M., Haines, J., Story, M., & Eisenberg, M. E. (2007). Why does dieting predict weight gain in adolescents? Findings from Project EAT-II: A 5-year longitudinal study. *Journal of the American Dietetic Association, 107*, 448–455.

Noakes, M., Foster, P. R., Keogh, J. B., & Clifton, P. M. (2004). Meal replacements are as effective as structured weight-loss diets for treating obesity in adults with features of metabolic syndrome. *The Journal of Nutrition, 134*, 1894–1899.

Paul-Ebhohimhen, V., & Avenell, A. (2008). Systematic review of the use of financial incentives in treatments for obesity and overweight. *Obesity Reviews, 9*, 355–367.

Perri, M. G., & Corsica, J. A. (2002). Improving the maintenance of weight lost in behavioral treatment of obesity. In T. A. Wadden & A. J. Stunkard (Eds.), *Handbook of obesity treatment* (pp. 357–379). New York, NY: Guilford Press.

Picot, J., Jones, J., Colquitt, J. L., Gospodarevskaya, E., Loveman, E., Baxter, L., Clegg, A. J. (2009). The clinical effectiveness and cost-effectiveness of bariatric (weight loss) surgery for obesity: A systematic review and economic evaluation. *Health Technology Assessment, 13*(41), 1–190.

Salahi, L. (2011). *Weight loss drugs: Public citizen calls for ban on Alli, Xenical.* Retrieved April 21, 2011, from http://abcnews.go.com/Health/w_DietAndFitness/weight-loss-drugs-consumer-watchdog-calls-ban-alli/story?id=13376523

Senturk, T., Ozdabakoglu, O., & Baran, I. (2008). Acute myocardial infarction associated with use of herbal medication. *Clinical Research in Cardiology, 97*, 784–786.

Seow-Choen, F. (2009). The physiology of colonic hydrotherapy. *Colorectal Disease, 11*, 686–688.

Sjostrom, L., Lindroos, A. K., Peltonen, M., Torgerson, J., Bouchard, C., Carlsson B., ... Wedel, H. (2004). Lifestyle, diabetes, and cardiovascular risk factors 10 years after bariatric surgery. *New England Journal of Medicine, 351*, 2683–2693.

Spear, B. A., Barlow, S. E., Ervin, C., Ludwig, D. S., Saelens, B. E., Schetzina, K. E., Taveras, E. M. (2007). Recommendations for treatment of child and adolescent overweight and obesity. *Pediatrics, 120*, S254–S288.

Tsai, A. G., & Wadden, T. A. (2005). Systematic review: An evaluation of major commercial weight loss programs in the United States. *Annals of Internal Medicine, 142,* 56–66.

Tsai, A. G., & Wadden, T. A. (2006). The evolution of low-calories diets: An update and meta-analysis. *Obesity, 14,* 1283–1293.

Wadden, T. A., Crerand, C. E., & Brock, J. (2005). Behavioral treatment of obesity. *Psychiatric Clinics of North America, 28,* 151–170.

Wadden, T. A., Womble, L. G., Sarwer, D. B., Berkowitz, R. I., Clark, V. L., & Foster, G. D. (2003). Great expectations: "I'm losing 25% of my weight no matter what you say." *Journal of Consulting and Clinical Psychology, 71,* 1084–1089.

Weiss, E. C., Galuska, D. A., Khan, L. K., Gillespie, C., & Serdula, M. K. (2007). Weight regain in U.S. adults who experienced sustained weight loss, 1999–2002. *American Journal of Preventive Medicine, 33,* 34–40.

Weiss, E. C., Galuska, D. A., Khan, L. K., & Serdula, M. K. (2006). Weight-control practices among U.S. adults, 2001–2002. *American Journal of Preventive Medicine, 31,* 18–24.

Wing, R. R. (2002). Behavioral weight control. In T. A. Wadden & A. J. Stunkard (Eds.), *Handbook of obesity treatment* (pp. 301–316). New York, NY: Guilford Press.

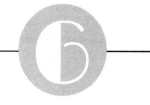

Prevention of Obesity

n the previous chapter, you learned how difficult it is to treat obesity effectively. Aside from surgical approaches, the long-term success rates of obesity treatments are pretty grim. If you were administering a program to people being released from prison designed to reduce the chances they will be incarcerated again, and 95% of them ended up back in prison within five years, you might say we need to try a different approach.[1] Given the somber statistics on long-term weight loss following obesity treatment, many have called for a different approach to this problem. If obesity is so incredibly hard to treat effectively, then maybe we need to be focusing on not letting people become obese in the first place! But where should prevention start? How do you prevent large groups of people from becoming obese?

TYPES OF PREVENTION

There are three categories of prevention: primary, secondary, and tertiary. Primary prevention means that you are targeting the entire population. If we are trying to prevent skin cancer, then we want absolutely *everyone* to start wearing sunscreen at all times. Secondary prevention focuses on populations who are "at risk." So, instead of asking everyone to wear sunscreen, we might ask only those people who have a family history of skin cancer to lather on the zinc oxide, or maybe offer free sunscreen samples to everyone who lives near the beach. Tertiary prevention programs target those who are already on track to develop the disease (or are in the early stages of it) but haven't yet experienced any bad consequences. So, we would focus on finding people who had some sort of early-stage skin cancer and make sure they stay out of the sun so that the malignancy doesn't grow and get worse. Tertiary prevention is similar to treatment, in that we are looking at people who already have a disease and trying to prevent future problems or symptoms.

Applied to obesity, you can see that primary prevention efforts would focus on everyone, regardless of their weight status, family history, or risk factors. Secondary prevention efforts might focus on children whose parents are obese, or individuals who are overweight, or communities made up of mostly fast-food restaurants, or any subpopulation that might be considered at higher risk for developing obesity. Tertiary prevention might focus on preventing diabetes or heart disease in already obese individuals. Since most tertiary prevention efforts would likely entail weight loss, or some sort of diet and physical activity intervention that we have described in the previous chapter, we are going to stick to primary and secondary prevention (for the most part) for the remainder of this chapter.

There are pros and cons to each approach. If you design a primary prevention program directed at the whole population, then you stand to reach the largest number of people. However, maybe that would be a waste of resources because a third of your population may not need any assistance in preventing weight gain. They would be just fine on their own. With a secondary prevention program, you could devote all your resources to a subpopulation in greatest need. However, you would likely exclude a large number of people who could benefit from your program because they might not meet whatever definition you set for "at risk." There are also issues of stigmatization when you target specific groups of people. We will discuss this topic further, particularly in reference to children and adolescents.

Speaking of children and adolescents…one of the first steps in prevention is deciding when to intervene. Do we try to prevent obesity in utero? During infancy? Early childhood? When adolescents leave for college? Since obesity is so difficult to reverse, most prevention research has focused on preventing inappropriate weight gain in children and adolescents. If you were trying to design a program for all children and adolescents in the United States, a logical place to find them would be schools.

SCHOOL-BASED PROGRAMS

Since the vast majority of children in the United States spend about half of their waking hours in school, schools have been a natural target for primary and secondary obesity prevention interventions. Youth spend more time in school than any other place outside their home, so it makes sense that programs targeting children and adolescents would be designed to reach children through their schools. Beyond just being an easy place to find children, school environments can significantly influence the likelihood of obesity based on the availability of healthy food options and opportunities for physical activity.

Children eat one or two meals in school each day (and additional snacks from vending machines). Unfortunately, the majority of food served in U.S. schools is pretty unhealthy (Story, Nanney, & Schwartz, 2009). One study surveyed the food available in several high schools and categorized the food options as "red" (providing little nutritional value and high levels of calories; e.g., chips, fries, sugar-sweetened beverages), "yellow" (foods that should be eaten in moderation, but provide some nutrition; e.g., bagels, rolls, chef salads), and "green" (foods that should be eaten often; fruits and vegetables, water, low-fat milk and yogurt). For foods served in the National School Lunch Program (NSLP), 23% of the food offered fell in the red category, 44% fell in the yellow category, and 33% fell in the green category. For competitive foods (i.e., food not part of NSLP and typically unregulated by the government for quality or nutritional standards, such as foods found in vending machines), 61% fell in the red category, 17% in the yellow, and 22% in the green category (Snelling, Korba, & Burkey, 2007). A survey in 2006 revealed that 62% of middle schools and 86% of high schools had at least one vending machine that sold snacks or beverages, most frequently soda and salty, high fat snacks (O'Toole, Anderson, Miller, & Guthrie, 2007). In terms of physical activity, only 4% of elementary schools, 8% of middle schools, and 2% of high schools provide daily physical education, with 22% of schools not requiring it at all (Lee, Burgeson, Fulton, & Spain, 2007). Students are getting less physical activity before and after school as well; less than 13% of students walked or biked to school in 2004, compared with more than 50% in 1969 (Kweon, Shin, Folzenlogen, & Kim, 2007).

Most school-based interventions aimed at preventing obesity have focused on a few key areas: improving the food offered in school, increasing opportunities for physical activity (during, before, and after school), health and nutrition education curricula, and screening youth for overweight and obesity.

Improving School Foods

There are many different ways to improve the food available in schools.

- Mandating that school lunches, vending machines, and a la carte foods meet certain criteria for calories, fat, and/or salt. These kinds of policy changes can occur at the school level (though most individual schools do not have control over their food offerings), district level, state level, or federal level.
- Limiting the availability of unhealthy foods by closing vending machines during certain hours, taking soda out of schools, preventing students from leaving campus during lunch, etc. Again, these decisions are often not under the control of individual schools, but policies can be changed at a variety of levels. Getting soda out of schools was a major initiative of several public health advocacy organizations, including the William J. Clinton Foundation (it helps to have a former President backing a cause). Several states successfully mandated that soda be removed from schools, and enough pressure accumulated that the largest soda companies in the United States (including Coca-Cola and Pepsi) agreed to voluntarily remove high-calorie sodas from schools by 2009. Of course, these companies still sell diet soda, flavored waters, and sports drinks, so their bottom lines were hardly affected by the change.
- Farm-to-school programs involve having local farms provide schools with fresh produce, and typically also include visits to the farms and having farmers speak to students in the classroom. School gardens allow students to grow their own fruits and vegetables, and typically include an educational component (in terms of educating students about food systems, but it may also be related to biology or nutrition curricula). Both farm-to-school and school garden programs have not been rigorously evaluated. Although these kinds of programs are not likely to have any significant impact on obesity

rates, such programs can help provide schools with fruits and vegetables they may not otherwise be able to purchase.

- "Central kitchens" are food production sites that provide food to all the schools in a city, county, or district. Instead of having each school be responsible for food preparation (which often just involves warming up prepackaged meals), a central kitchen prepares meals and delivers food to schools. The central kitchen may obtain ingredients from local farms or partner with local businesses and institutions (e.g., restaurants, grocers, culinary schools), with the goal of creating fresh, healthy meals from scratch. Cooking healthy foods from scratch is typically impossible for individual schools, which may be equipped only with several microwaves to reheat food and lack the adequately trained food service staff to create and cook healthy items. This type of intervention also has not yet been evaluated. As with many of the options described above, this particular program may not have a measurable impact on obesity rates, but is likely beneficial in that it improves the quality of food served in school settings.

Physical Activity

As we mentioned previously, schools rarely provide children with daily opportunities for physical activity; and if they do, the activities are of short duration and low intensity. In addition, we have personally observed schools punishing individual students or classrooms for misbehavior by removing the only 10-minute recess of the day, or forcing low performing students to replace physical education or recess with more instruction time. As a result, many school-based obesity prevention programs have focused on getting students to participate in more physical activity before, during, and after school. These efforts can include a number of different approaches:

- Requiring students to participate in gym class on a daily (or at least several times per week) basis. As with the school food

policies mentioned above, policies regarding physical education can be made at a variety of levels but are often not under
the control of the individual school.

- Encouraging participation in after-school sports programs, and/or providing a variety of after-school sports
opportunities.
- Encouraging students to reduce television (TV) watching and
video gaming (and other sedentary activities).
- Incorporating a 15-minute activity break between classes.
- Allowing students to use playgrounds, gyms, tracks, basket-
ball courts, etc. during recess or lunch periods.
- Encouraging students to walk or bike to and from school.
These "Safe-Routes-to-School" and "Walking School Bus"
programs have been effective in boosting the number of
students who walk or bike to school (Davison, Werder, &
Lawson, 2008).

Most of these physical activity interventions have not
been evaluated over the long term, and shorter-term studies
have reported mixed findings. A recent meta-analysis reported
that physical activity interventions in schools generally had
no impact on body mass index (BMI) (Harris, Kuramoto,
Schulzer, & Retallack, 2009). However, another recent review
of 26 studies reported that there were a number of positive
outcomes to physical activity interventions in schools, including higher levels of physical activity (duh), less TV viewing,
better physical fitness, and improved cholesterol (Dobbins,
De Corby, Robeson, Husson, & Tirillis, 2009). Since most of
the studies were relatively short term (two years or less), it is
not surprising that there would be no significant impact on
BMI, but positive impacts on a variety of other more immediate outcomes. It is also possible that these programs included
students who were not yet overweight or obese, leading to no
significant change in BMI overall. Positive effects on physical
activity are encouraging because developing good habits early
may help prevent obesity later in life.

Health and Nutrition Education

Many obesity prevention programs have looked at adding health, nutrition, and physical education courses to the school day. Supporters of such programs believe that if we educate children about their overall health, and how nutrition and physical activity can result in improvements in health, then we will end up with a whole generation of healthier individuals. After all, do we expect children to just know the difference between saturated and poly- or monounsaturated fats, or the various sources of sodium and the effect they have on health? Although many schools already require that nutrition or health be taught, the amount of time devoted to these subjects is, quite candidly, pathetic. Elementary schools spend less than 3.5 hours and middle and high schools spend less than 5 hours per year on these topics (Story et al., 2009). It is hard to imagine how any child or adolescent is going to take away anything meaningful from these 5 hours of classes when the other 8,755 hours of the year are spent doing other things, such as watching TV, sleeping, being bombarded with advertisements for video games and unhealthy snacks, etc. Five hours per year simply cannot compete with the thousands of hours per year of unhealthy "education" that children receive just through the course of their daily lives. After all, these five hours per year are dwarfed by the almost five hours per day spent watching TV for the average American (The Nielsen Company, 2011). Yikes.

BMI Monitoring/Reporting

As we mentioned in the previous chapter, only 20% to 50% of overweight children are actually identified as being overweight or obese, and even fewer get treatment (Benson, Baer, & Kaelber, 2009; Louthan et al., 2005). One initiative that has been proposed is to screen children and teens for obesity in schools, similar to the hearing and vision screenings that already take place. Confidential "report cards" are then sent home to parents describing the students' weight status. The idea is that this information can empower parents (and students) to either seek treatment or to initiate some behavior changes at home (Nihiser et al., 2007). After all, the first step in solving a problem is recognizing that a problem exists. Some schools also collect BMI data on students for surveillance purposes, where information is anonymous and used to track whether certain school policies (or local or state policies) are effective in reducing rates of obesity for the school, district, or state as a whole.

Arkansas passed legislation in 2003 mandating that all public schools collect BMI measurements. Several other states have followed suit to allow BMI screening and reporting in schools. Many people criticized this approach, saying that it could lead to stigmatization and teasing of obese and overweight children, pressure from parents to diet, an increase in eating disorders, and violations of privacy. Results of evaluations of the Arkansas legislation have suggested that obesity rates have not increased in the state since the screening was initiated in 2003 (Justus et al., 2007; Raczynski, Thompson, Phillips, Ryan, & Cleveland, 2009). Rates haven't decreased, but it is encouraging that they have not increased either, given that rates have increased elsewhere. Note, however, that the Arkansas legislation included a number of other components, such as restricting vending machine access, so we can't attribute the plateau in obesity rates solely to the BMI screening.

Additionally, the evaluations have shown that the criticisms of the legislation were largely unfounded. The vast majority of parents are supportive of the effort, teasing and eating disorders have not increased, and neither have unhealthy dietary practices (Kubik, Story, & Rieland, 2007; Raczynski et al., 2009). Unfortunately, it is commonplace for any new trend or idea to be challenged by someone. For example, the Beatles were initially rejected by Decca Records, who famously noted, "guitar groups are on the way out." Oops. Opposition to new ideas does not preclude the potential for success.

One important thing to note with respect to screening programs is that they are not exactly a prevention program in and of themselves. For example, suppose scientists had developed a screening test for Alzheimer's disease. People would have their cheeks swabbed at their doctors' offices and be told whether or not they would develop Alzheimer's. We could widely implement this test to screen the population for Alzheimer's, but it would be completely useless in preventing the disease. In fact, it might actually be harmful because people would be told (and some incorrectly so) that they will develop a devastating disease that they cannot prevent; only (possibly) delay its onset. Further, the cost of implementing a wide-scale screening program would be considerable.

In other words, we have to make sure that if we provide people with information about their weight or their children's weight, and spend valuable dollars in doing so, the information can and will be useful. For many years, it was unclear whether providing BMI information to parents was worth the effort. After all, we have discussed the limitations of weight-loss treatment in Chapter 5. However, recently, the U.S. Preventive Services Task Force (USPSTF) has recommended that children and adolescents be screened for obesity (USPSTF, 2010). The USPSTF concluded that screening programs can be effective when children and teens are referred to comprehensive weight management programs involving counseling, behavior modification, diet, and physical activity (that typically also involves the child's family). These recommendations do not specify that children should be screened in schools, just that screening can be useful overall. If screening is to be performed in a school setting, then parents also need some way of obtaining the appropriate referrals for treatment. Schools can include information on community resources, or suggest that parents discuss treatment options with a pediatrician. In Arkansas, a survey of pediatricians reported that 57% had a parent bring in a BMI report card to discuss, suggesting that the letters can inspire parents to engage in conversations about their children's weights with health care professionals (Raczynski et al., 2009). It's not perfect—but it's a start.

Preschool Interventions

The school-based interventions described above have primarily been implemented in elementary, middle, or high schools. It is a completely open question, however, as to when it is best to intervene in a child's life—perhaps it is even earlier, in the preschool years. After all, the prevalence of obesity among preschoolers has risen in dramatic fashion in recent years, just as it has for the rest of the population. Disparities in obesity rates between racial and ethnic subgroups are apparent by age four (Anderson & Whitaker, 2009). So maybe we are already too late if we intervene with only K through 12 students.

There are very few obesity prevention programs that have been evaluated for preschool-aged children, and most have shown mixed results (Saunders, 2007). Some interventions have included things such as encouraging breastfeeding among mothers. Others have included some of the school-based activities described above, such as encouraging physical activity. Others still have focused on maternal (or paternal) feeding practices, parenting practices and health behaviors, and reducing TV watching. The studies on these initiatives have been pretty limited. At this point, we really don't know what works at all, let alone what works best for the preschool population. The only conclusions we can draw are that some things are worth encouraging in and of themselves, such as higher levels of physical activity and healthier diets (i.e., do not feed your 2-year-old Coca-Cola in his or her bottle), even if it doesn't lead to a significant change in BMI according to the existing research. Additionally, programs that address many different components (i.e., diet, activity, parent skills and behaviors, the home environment) are likely to be more effective than interventions that focus on only one or two components (Bluford, Sherry, & Scanlon, 2007). Programs promoting healthy behaviors among preschoolers may lead to lower rates of obesity over time, but we need a lot more research in this area before we can determine what type of prevention program works best in this age group.

Overcoming Barriers to Success in the School Setting

School-based interventions must overcome the challenges of competing priorities in the school setting (e.g., academics) combined with limited staff and administrative resources available for additional curricula and training related to nutrition, health, or physical education. In the age of state standardized testing, many schools and their administrators do not want to devote any time to physical education, health classes, or nutrition education, particularly when school funding and jobs depend on the results of math and science assessments. However, up to an hour of daily physical activity can be added to a school curriculum without having a negative impact on students' academic performance (Trudeau & Shephard, 2008). In fact, there is no disputing that physical activity is good for students' learning.

Additionally, policies to improve the availability of healthy foods (generally by limiting unhealthy food offerings in vending machines, school lunch programs, and a la carte lines) often face opposition because of the fear of decreased revenues. The salty, fatty, high-calorie snacks sell! You might imagine that restocking vending machines with apples and carrots would put a damper on sales. However, research has suggested that the food offered in schools can be made more healthful without adversely effecting school revenues (Story et al., 2009). Generally, small changes such as replacing whole milk with skim or low-fat milk, or fried chips with baked chips, go over pretty well and sometimes even go unnoticed.

School lunch programs are a little more complicated when it comes down to finances. Schools are reimbursed by the federal government for the "free" meals they provide to students. The reimbursement rate is about $2.50 per meal (Story et al.,

2009), give or take a few cents. Do you think you could make a healthy meal for $2.50? This rate is supposed to cover the costs of buying the food, transporting it to the school, and the salaries of the school food service staff who prepare the food. When you break it down, it seems like a pretty impossible task to cover all of that with just $2.50 per meal, let alone create something healthy that students will want to eat. (Remember what we said about how healthier food costs more in Chapter 2?)

In December 2010, President Barack Obama signed the federal Healthy, Hunger-Free Kids Act of 2010, with the intent to develop children's interest in consuming fruits and vegetables and engaging in healthier lifestyles. The bill requires schools to make healthier choices available to students, and offers financial incentives in the amount of 6 cents per meal for those that do well at meeting nutritional standards. Naturally, this was supported by his wife, Michelle Obama, who has actively pursued methods of reducing childhood obesity. However, the costs associated with improving meals in some districts may be as much as 20 cents or more, meaning a loss of 14 cents per meal. It seems small, but it adds up. In a time when schools are making more and more cuts based on dwindling budgets, it comes as no surprise that such incentives are met with some trepidation. This bill would also force students not receiving free or reduced lunches to pay more—these families likely have something to say about that.

Interventions in Primary Care and Other Settings

The BMI screening and reporting efforts we described above could also take place in a primary care setting. In fact, it may be that pediatricians and family practice doctors are better equipped to conduct BMI screening than schools, as physicians (presumably) are better able to make the appropriate referrals for comprehensive weight management treatment, or even to provide some weight management counseling to their patients. Other prevention interventions have focused on training health care providers to deal more effectively with overweight and obese patients. However, The Community Preventive Services Task Force has found insufficient evidence to recommend provider-oriented prevention approaches (Community Preventive Services, 2010).

Other settings, such as maternal and child health clinics, Head Start offices, or offices for the Women, Infants and Children (WIC) program, have been suggested as good places to reach children (and their parents) to deliver obesity prevention programs. These programs could include BMI screening and reporting, referrals for weight management treatment, dietary counseling, physical activity programs, or any combination of these and other activities. Although some small programs have been attempted, nothing to date has been widely implemented in any of these settings.

SUMMARY: OBESITY PREVENTION IN CHILDREN AND ADOLESCENTS

Those of us in the research world often turn to meta-analyses and huge systematic reviews to get a (somewhat) authoritative answer to whether a particular program or intervention is effective. The systematic reviews completed thus far on obesity prevention programs in children have suggested that they are a mixed bag. First, most of the studies are pretty short term (one year or less), and as we know from the last chapter, the real test in weight loss is whether it is sustained over the long term. Second, they use a variety of different methods and target populations, so it is hard to draw any conclusions without replicated findings. Essentially, it is as if you have a bag of apples, oranges, pears, and grapes, and someone asks you to describe what the contents of the bag taste like overall. It is hard to distill a bunch of different things into one result or finding. Generally speaking, however, we can say:

1. Obesity prevention programs that involve dietary or physical activity interventions result in improvements to diet and physical activity levels, at least for the short term (that's good, but expected; Summerbell et al., 2005).
2. Most programs have no effect on BMI, or a small effect at best (that's not good, but also expected; Brown & Summerbell, 2009; Katz, O'Connell, Njike, Yeh, & Nawaz, 2008; Summerbell et al., 2005).
3. School-based interventions that combine a variety of approaches (i.e., programs that target both diet and physical activity, as well as modify the school environment) may help prevent children from becoming overweight or obese (Brown & Summerbell, 2009; Katz et al., 2008), but the results so far are pretty underwhelming.

There are several reasons we might not expect to see any impact on BMI from these programs. First, most studies of prevention programs aren't very long. It takes a relatively short period of time to have an effect on diet and activity, but it takes a long time for those small changes to result in a big enough shift in energy balance to change BMI for a whole population of children. Most studies are simply not long enough to demonstrate any measurable effect on obesity rates.

Second, back to the issue of primary versus secondary prevention, most studies target a whole school full of children (or several schools). The students in these schools comprise underweight children, normal weight children, overweight children, and obese children. As we discussed above, it may be that two thirds of the children are going to be under- or normal weight no matter what, so the prevention programs will likely have no measurable impact on them. When you include everyone, the effects can get somewhat muddled or diluted. At this point in time, we simply do not know whether it would be more effective to target children who are "at risk" or include everyone. Related to this issue is that of the appropriate target age group. Should we focus on preschoolers? Middle schoolers? If we focus on high school students, is it too late? It is unclear what age group(s) should be targeted if we are going to maximize the effectiveness of obesity prevention efforts.

Third (and this is probably the most important reason), obesity is caused by hundreds, if not thousands of different factors. Why on earth would we expect that changing just one or two things (e.g., school food, physical education classes, etc.) would have any measurable effect on BMI? Probably, the best we can hope for is that we would be able to detect meaningful changes in diet and activity levels (which are good for their own sake), and that these changes *may* result in fewer children becoming overweight or obese over time. However, it is likely that *several* (read: a dozen, two dozen, or many more) different interventions need to be implemented concurrently in order to make any sort of measurable dent in the obesity epidemic.

WORKPLACE INTERVENTIONS

If you would go to schools to locate children, where would you go to locate adults to deliver obesity prevention programs? Likely their workplace. Employed adults spend a great deal of time at work. Additionally, employers have an incentive to maintain a healthy workforce in order to reduce health care premiums and boost worker productivity. Workplace interventions can involve a variety of different strategies, similar to school-based prevention programs.

Education

Lectures, written materials, and other educational strategies designed to increase physical activity and improve diet can be provided to employees.

Counseling

Individual or group counseling can be used to promote behavior change. This can include skill-building activities, rewards, or reinforcements for healthy behaviors (e.g., walking 10,000 steps per day, or eating at least five vegetables per day). These counseling sessions may include coworkers, friends, or family members to provide social support. They can be run by health professionals, dieticians, or trained counselors.

Workplace Policies

Rules or procedures for employees can be changed to better promote health and health behaviors. For example, health insurance benefits can be changed to include coverage for weight-loss treatment or gym memberships. The workplace can also partner with local health clubs to provide discounted memberships. Additionally, workplaces may provide comprehensive health promotion programs to address things such as smoking cessation and stress management. Policies can also be changed to allow (and promote) ten-minute activity breaks throughout the day.

Changing the Workplace Environment

There are a number of ways workplaces can change the physical environment to make it more conducive to health. If there is a cafeteria, foods offered can be made healthier and/or nutrition information can be provided where employees can see it before purchasing lunch. Place signs encouraging employees to make healthier choices near the counters. Nutrition information can be provided at vending machines, and healthier items can be stocked. Point-of-decision signs and prompts can be used to encourage healthy food choices and physical activity. For example, place a large sign by the stairs that says "Take the stairs, it's good for your health!" Even a small prompt like that can have a dramatic effect on the number of people who use the stairs

(Soler et al., 2010). More intensive interventions might involve having a gym on site for employees, or installing better lighting in staircases so people are more likely to use them.

Barriers to Success in the Workplace

These workplace interventions cost about $1.44 to $4.16 per pound of body weight lost (Anderson et al., 2009). Many workplaces may simply not have the capacity to offer gym memberships, hire a counselor to deliver a group-based behavior modification program, or overhaul the food available in the cafeteria. Additionally, one of the limitations of most of the studies of workplace interventions is that they were conducted primarily in white-collar offices. It is unclear whether workplace interventions would be successful (even by the modest standard of a two-pound weight loss) in other types of environments where employees are performing manual labor, or are required to travel (e.g., truck drivers, pilots), or in service-oriented worksites (e.g., retail stores, restaurants, etc.), or in blue-collar occupations. Once again, the research simply cannot tell us much yet. If you're looking for a dissertation topic, you're welcome.

BMI Screening

Just as with children, we learned that many adults incorrectly perceive their own weight. About one in three normal-weight adults, 38% of overweight adults, and 8% of obese adults incorrectly categorize their own weight (Dorsey, Eberhardt, & Ogden, 2009). Logically, there may be value in informing adults of their weight status, so that they can be referred to (or seek out) treatment. The USPSTF (2003) recommends that primary care physicians screen all adults for obesity and refer obese adults to intensive behavioral interventions (i.e., programs that combine nutrition education and counseling, physical activity, and behavior modification) to promote long-term weight loss. This particular recommendation is an example of tertiary prevention, where obese adults are referred for intensive treatment in order to stave off weight-related health complications. However, there may be some benefit to overweight or normal-weight individuals at risk of weight gain receiving feedback from their physicians about their weight. They may engage in self-initiated weight-management regimens, or seek counseling from their physicians or other programs. In this case, screening could serve as a secondary prevention effort. Then again, there are not any evaluations of screening programs for adults indicating the effectiveness of this type of intervention.

Not everyone agrees with the recommendation of the USPSTF (e.g., Wilson & McAlpine, 2006). In order for screening to be considered an effective intervention, several things have to be true: (1) the condition is prevalent (certainly true for obesity); (2) you have an accurate way of diagnosing the condition (we discussed the limitations of BMI in Chapter 1); (3) screening poses minimal risk (measuring BMI is pretty mundane); and (4) knowing about the condition early leads to effective treatment for the condition (Wilson & McAlpine, 2006). This last point is probably the most debatable with respect to obesity screening, as we discussed in Chapter 5. If we use a very loose definition of "effective," then there are treatment programs that can be effective in producing sustained weight losses of a few pounds. However, these treatment studies typically enroll dream participants—people with no related health problems, who are highly motivated, and who responded to ads in the paper describing the weight-loss study. The average person visiting their primary care doctor is not the ideal research participant. They may have zero motivation to engage in the intensive behavioral weight-loss treatment program prescribed by their physician, even after finding out that they are obese. If we implement a screening program, and most obese people either choose not to follow-through with their physician's recommendations for treatment, or can't because it would be too expensive and not covered by insurance, or treatment is not successful for them—what good have we done? We have simply wasted resources in implementing the program, with no measurable benefit to show for it.

SUMMARY OF OBESITY PREVENTION PROGRAMS IN ADULTS

Worksite health promotion programs have been found to be moderately successful at reducing BMI among employees. Of course, this relies on your definition of "success." Workplace interventions aimed at increasing physical activity and diet (or both) result in an average weight loss of 2.8 pounds over the course of six months to one year, or a reduction in BMI of 0.47 kg/m² (Anderson et al., 2009). This outcome sounds good, as small weight losses mean that we are preventing weight gain, right? However, reporting results this way can be misleading. Maybe only normal-weight individuals lose three pounds and everyone else is unaffected. Or obese individuals lose five pounds, but they are still obese. It would probably be more helpful to know what percentage of employees became obese over time, or if this proportion declined. However, most studies do not report results in this manner. Because of the modest weight losses reported in several studies, workplace obesity prevention programs have been recommended by the Community Preventive Services Task Force (Task Force on Community Preventive Services, 2009). Ultimately, we need some more research to be done before we can definitively say that this type of program is an effective (and cost-effective) obesity prevention measure, with particular emphasis on whether weight was sustained for the long term.

Not much evidence supports other types of obesity prevention interventions in adults (Lemmens, Oenema, Klepp, Henriksen, & Brug, 2008). The other types of prevention programs that have been evaluated typically involve lifestyle counseling that consists of a combination of diet and physical activity, as well as an educational component. Some interventions are less intensive, involving monthly newsletters to educate people on diet and physical activity, or telephone or Web-based programs. A systematic review of interventions to prevent weight gain in adults reported that 11 out of 39 studies were effective (resulting in a two-year or longer weight loss of approximately 1 to 25 pounds; Brown et al., 2009). The interventions included in this review included: a low-fat diet reducing caloric intake by 600 calories per day (with and without meal replacements), low-calorie diets, Weight Watchers, low-fat diets, diets with behavior therapy, diets with exercise, diets without exercise, and behavior therapy alone. Do these sound familiar? They should. They were all covered in Chapter 5 when we discussed treatment (did you pass our test?). These could really be classified as tertiary prevention interventions in that they targeted moderately obese individuals (BMI less than 35 kg/m^2) with the intent to prevent subsequent weight gain and reduce the likelihood that they would develop obesity-related health problems. It is not exactly encouraging that only 28% of the studies showed any success, especially when the bar for "success" is so low.

Community Approaches

You might have noticed that the prevention interventions we have discussed thus far are individually or small group focused. Some of the strategies, such as modifying school or workplace environments, have the potential to affect larger groups of people, but most of the strategies are targeted at relatively small groups of individuals. They include offering education, counseling, referrals for treatment, etc. Of course, if these strategies were implemented across all the schools and workplaces in the United States, they could have a tremendous impact. However, in most of the interventions described above, the burden of change rests on the individual. Parents are expected to change their children's eating and activity behavior (and their own), employees are expected to follow diet and exercise programs, and patients are expected to follow up on physician referrals and obtain weight-loss treatment. This seems like a lot to expect from two thirds of our population. If you want to change the behavior of more than 200 million people, do you think the most effective approach is to tell them one-by-one to eat healthier, or simply to tell them that they are, in fact, overweight?

A different approach would be to change aspects of our communities and environments in ways that encourage healthier behaviors. When we discussed causes of obesity in Chapter 2, we described how factors at various levels interact to cause obesity. Individual-level factors are important, but they themselves are often determined by higher-level factors related to our communities, economies, and policies. For example, the food that we eat on a weekly basis is affected by not only our individual preferences and knowledge but also where we live and what food sources are nearby, or how much healthy food costs in comparison to the fast-food restaurant down the street. How much physical activity we get is influenced by things such as having a gym or park nearby, living within walking distance of school or work, or having sidewalks in our neighborhoods.

Suppose an entire town had sewer holes without covers throughout the city. Over time, research found that the majority of people had fallen in a sewer hole at one point, sustaining injury requiring medical treatment. You could try to educate people about the sewer holes, give them maps of the sewer holes to carry around, provide incentives to people who go the longest period without falling in one, teach people how to respond if they happened to fall in one, target groups that walk a lot or are visually impaired and can't see the holes, and so forth; but wouldn't it make more sense to just cover the sewer holes?

Changing the Built Environment

There are numerous manmade environmental structures, collectively known as the "built environment," (Booth, Pinkston, & Poston, 2005) that could be changed to facilitate healthier eating patterns and increase physical activity. The built environment essentially refers to how our communities are built. It includes things such as the buildings we live, work, or go to school in; sidewalks, roads, and bike paths; playgrounds and parks; where we shop, etc. These components can be modified in various ways to make it more likely that residents engage in physical activity or healthier eating.

- Communities can ensure that residents have the ability to walk or bike to work, school, or shopping areas by creating sidewalks and bike paths. Existing paths can be made safer through better lighting, policing, or traffic calming endeavors. Residents won't walk or bike places if everything is far away, so communities can be designed to ensure that people have everything they need close by: grocery stores and shopping areas should be located near residential areas (this is called "mixed land use").
- Urban areas can adopt "smart growth" policies, which limit urban sprawl (where cities and suburbs are spread over so much area it makes it necessary to drive long distances to get anywhere you need to go) and make it easier for residents to commute by walking or biking. These smart growth policies are beneficial in terms of facilitating physical activity among residents through providing opportunities for active transportation, but they also are worth doing for environmental reasons. Fewer cars, more public transportation options, and a greater proportion of people walking or biking means less smog and greenhouse gas emissions.
- Zoning code restrictions can be used to limit the number of restaurants and convenience stores in specified areas, such as within a certain distance of schools. Zoning codes are rules set by local governments specifying what kind of buildings, and how many of them, can exist in a certain location (in terms of the structure of the building as well as the function or use). For example, the zoning code for a city may stipulate that a certain building (or area) be used for residential

purposes, while another is to be used for commercial purposes. Zoning policies can also specify those commercial purposes. For example, the zoning code can prohibit fast-food restaurants from existing in a given area. It can also stipulate that small grocery stores stock a certain amount of healthy food (or limit unhealthy items) in order to operate at a particular location.

Changing the Food Environment

Similar to the built environment, the "food environment" refers to the food sources within our communities. Neighborhood or community food environments comprise "the number, type, location, and accessibility of food outlets such as grocery stores, fast-food restaurants, and full-service restaurants" (Story, Kaphingst, Robinson-O'Brien, & Glanz, 2008, p. 265). In other words, the food stores, restaurants, markets, mobile food stands, gardens, and farms, in a given area. The food environment can be altered using some of the tools described above, such as changes to zoning codes. There are several other ways that communities could improve the food environment in order to foster healthier eating.

- Local governments can provide incentives (e.g., tax breaks) to stores providing healthy foods or to supermarkets in order open in a given locality (Gostin, 2007). Barriers to opening supermarkets or farmer's markets can be removed (i.e., features of the existing zoning code sometimes serve to block opportunities to open markets). Philadelphia has been at the forefront of this incentives approach, with their "Fresh Food Financing" effort. Grants, loans, and tax credits are provided to supermarkets that are willing to open outlets in underserved areas. These efforts have been expanded to other locations with help from an organization called "The Food Trust," and some funding from Michelle Obama's "Let's Move" campaign. These efforts have been successful in increasing the availability of fresh, healthy food in needy areas, and they have provided valuable jobs and economic benefits to those locations as well.

● Health communication and social marketing can be used to promote messages of health and health behavior. Of course, the money that food megacorporations spend on advertising dwarfs that spent on health-promoting messages, so relying on social marketing to promote healthy eating and activity can feel a bit like trying to swim up a waterfall. Public health simply cannot compete with the multibillion dollar coffers of the Coca-Colas and PepsiCos of the world. However, there are examples of marketing and health communication efforts that have at least garnered some significant attention, if not changed people's behavior. The New York City Health Department has received both good and bad press for its "Pouring on the Pounds" campaign, which depicted (in one of its ads) a man drinking a glass full of fat, in an effort to reduce New Yorkers' soda consumption.[2] You might be familiar with the social marketing and health communication efforts utilized in tobacco control (the "Truth" campaigns). These types of efforts have been found to be a potentially effective way to change behavior, though the evidence is mixed (Gordon, McDermott, Stead, & Angus, 2006).

● Partnerships with local food stores (typically small grocers or stores that tend to stock unhealthy convenience items) can be developed in order to increase the availability of healthy food in those stores. Stores may be offered incentives to stock fresh fruits and vegetables, and given materials or instructions to promote the purchase of these healthier items. For example, stores can put up nutrition labels indicating healthier choices, use signs and advertising, or host cooking demonstrations or taste tests to highlight a healthy food. It is important that there is sufficient demand in the community for healthy food items, or these kinds of programs will not be cost effective for the stores. If the stores stock healthy items, but no one buys them, then the stores take a loss. So these types of initiatives likely need to be combined with marketing efforts described above.

- Community gardens, urban gardens or farms, and mobile fruit and vegetable stands have been proposed (and implemented) as a means to increase the availability of fresh fruits and vegetables in underserved areas. The New York City Department of Health has implemented a "Green Carts" program that provides permits, microloans, and technical assistance to mobile fruit and vegetable trucks (funded through a grant from a charitable organization). The Department of Health also provides marketing and outreach to promote the program among residents.

Many local governments have used zoning to limit the number of restaurants and convenience stores in specified areas, or experimented with providing incentives to stores offering healthy foods to open in a given locality, or have modified the built environment to facilitate physical activity (Ashe, Jernigan, Kline, & Galaz, 2003). However, there are not many evaluations of the outcomes of these kinds of interventions.

Food Policy Councils

If you think of the various departments within your local government, you'll notice that there is no "Department of Food." There are typically departments of health, planning, transportation, education, management and budget, parks and recreation, housing, fire and rescue, finance, etc. Although the food environment is clearly influenced by many of these things, such as transportation and planning, government officials in those departments often do not consider how their decisions may impact the availability of food in the community. Not to mention, there are many key players in the private sector that influence the food environment as well, but who may not communicate with public officials. Food policy councils have been established in a number of locations in order to address these gaps. They consist of a group of various stakeholders from different agencies and industries. They may include government officials, local business owners, community representatives, educators, and farmers. The food policy council serves as a means to get all these individuals with different interests and backgrounds to the same table in order to find agreeable solutions to various problems with the local food system.

There is no evidence to date demonstrating the effect of having a food policy council on the health of residents (or on other outcomes, such as food access or economic development; Harper, Shattuck, Holt-Gimenez, Alkon, & Lambrick, 2009). However, it is encouraging that governments in many locations are at least engaging in discussions of food-related issues through food policy councils, as food has largely been left out of the decision-making process. At the very least, food issues are deemed worthy of consideration and no longer an afterthought of other policies serving alternative interests.

Overcoming Barriers to Success at the Community Level

In order to be effective, community or environmental interventions will need to increase opportunities for healthy eating and activity *and* decrease opportunities for unhealthy dietary and sedentary activity choices; the reason being that if you simply offer someone some broccoli, but do not decrease their access to French fries, then that person is likely still going to choose the French fries. You have to make the broccoli more appealing while simultaneously making the French fries less appealing (by making them cost more, or making someone travel further to get them, etc.). This presents a problem though, because the makers of French fries will surely be opposed to any interventions making French fries less attractive to people. So for policies such as zoning restrictions limiting the number of fast-food restaurants in a given area, there is going to be opposition from the fast-food industry and other libertarian or free-market followers. This opposition often takes the form of lawsuits, which tend to be extremely expensive and serve as a pretty good deterrent to attempting to restrict access to unhealthy foods.

Generally there is more support for adding things such as farmer's markets or urban gardens than there is for restricting things. When it comes to interventions that restrict unhealthy choices, it is much more difficult to build the political and social support necessary to get things done. The problem with programs adding things is that they cost money. Even in the best economic climate, local governments, agencies, or institutions may have tremendous difficulty raising the necessary funds to implement obesity prevention programs, such as providing incentives to supermarkets or building bike paths.

While many different interventions targeting the community environment have been implemented, few have been evaluated. Therefore, the effectiveness of these types of interventions in addressing obesity is unknown. Hopefully as time goes on, evaluations of these interventions will be conducted and results made available. It is reasonable to assume, as with many of the previously described prevention programs, that these interventions could have a significant impact on the diets and physical activity levels of various communities. However, as with the other interventions, it is hard to imagine that any one program would have a measurable impact on obesity rates. Many different interventions will have to be implemented concurrently in order to make a visible dent in obesity rates, but you have to start somewhere.

POLICY APPROACHES

Some of the community-based approaches actually involve changes in policy, such as changes to the zoning code or smart growth policies. There are a number of other policy approaches that have been proposed. Although many of these policies could be implemented at the local or community level, they could be broadly applied at the state or federal level too, which is why they are described in this separate section.

Junk Food Taxes and Food Pricing

One method to decrease consumption of unhealthy foods is to tax them. If unhealthy foods such as soda, candy, and high-fat snack foods cost more, people would eat less of them. This method has been applied to tobacco and alcohol very successfully. One perk of a junk food tax is the revenue it could generate. A national penny-per-ounce tax on sugar-sweetened beverages could generate $79 billion in revenue over five years (Andreyeva, Chaloupka & Brownell, 2011). Taxes on food items would likely have to be pretty substantial in order to have an impact on food choice, generating even larger revenues (Kuchler, Tegene, & Harris, 2004). Revenues could be earmarked for obesity prevention and treatment programs, such as school or workplace interventions (e.g., those mentioned above), or to subsidize the sale of healthy foods (e.g., fruits and vegetables).

There is scientific support for the potential efficacy of a tax on certain foods in order to reduce consumption of those foods. Price is one of the primary determinants of food choice, along with taste, value, convenience, and, to a smaller extent, health (French, 2003; Glanz, Basil, Mailbach, Goldberg, & Snyder, 1998). Increasing the price of certain foods has been shown to be effective in reducing consumption (Epstein, Dearing, Roba, & Finkelstein, 2010; Epstein et al., 2006), and decreasing the price has been shown to be effective in increasing consumption of those items (French, 2003; Horgen & Brownell, 2002). A 20% price increase (through taxes) on sugar-sweetened beverages alone (e.g., soda, juice drinks, etc.) could result in a decrease in obesity prevalence among adults from 33.4% to 30.4% and among children from 16.6% to 13.7% (Smith, Lin, & Lee, 2010). The prevalence of overweight among adults could decrease from 66.9% to 62.4% and among children, from 32.3% to 27.0%.

Junk food taxes are hard to administer. How do you decide what foods qualify? Nutritionally, there may not be that much difference between an "energy bar" and a candy bar. Do you tax both, or just the Snickers and Milky Way because they are marketed as candy? It is very difficult to decide what foods to tax and how much. As a case in point, California previously instated a tax on snack foods, but repealed the policy in part because it was deemed too difficult to administer (Jacobson & Brownell, 2000). Although difficult to administer on a broad scale, several states have demonstrated limited success in implementing taxes on sodas and snack foods (Jacobson & Brownell, 2000).

This policy option is criticized for unfairly burdening the poor, since those of lower socioeconomic status (SES) consume a greater amount of unhealthy foods and would therefore be most burdened by a tax on those foods. However, those of lower SES may also benefit to a greater degree, because price is more important to lower SES people in making food decisions (French, 2003), and therefore price increases may lead to greater degrees of behavior change for low-income groups as compared with high-income groups who can already afford a healthy diet. Whether those of low SES or certain racial/ethnic groups would experience greater benefit from a junk food tax is unknown. Importantly, healthy food choices would have to be made more accessible and affordable. Otherwise, persons in poverty, still being unable to access or afford a healthy diet, will either be forced to pay more to maintain a diet of unhealthy foods or to go without food.

A coalition called Americans Against Food Taxes has strongly opposed junk food taxes, with ads that refer to such measures as raising the grocery costs for the middle-class families of America. Certainly, they make it seem as if middle-class families are *required* to buy junk food and soda, and thus will face increased grocery bills. Substituting the soda for some juice (or even cheaper—tap water), and exchanging the chips for a bag of carrots could actually reduce the overall grocery costs, not to mention medical bills in the future. Clever and manipulative advertising at its finest.

Some people have argued for subsidies of healthier foods instead of junk food taxes. No one likes taxes, and subsidies for fruits and vegetables are much more politically palatable. However, subsidies are not likely to be as effective as taxes (Epstein et al., 2010). Although providing subsidies for fruits and vegetables (and thereby reducing their cost) can increase the likelihood that people will buy them, people will still purchase cheap junk food. Taxing junk food such as soda and candy is a much more effective way of shifting dietary intake towards healthier options.

Food and Agriculture Policy

Agriculture policy is one factor that contributes to food price and availability. Agriculture policy could be changed to promote production of fruits and vegetables. Right now, some farmers actually face restrictions on planting fruits and vegetables. At the very least, these restrictions and barriers could be removed. Better yet, instead of providing incentives to plant corn and soybeans, we could subsidize the production of fruits and vegetables. These incentives could include making it easier for farmers who wish to plant fruits and vegetables to get loans (farming is an expensive business to run). Redirecting federal subsidies towards the production of fruits and vegetables may help to shift the overall pricing structure of foods to favor nutritious items.

The availability of nutritious food at the national level is insufficient to meet current dietary recommendations put forth by the U.S. government—assuming that all Americans actually followed those recommendations. Current estimates suggest that tremendous shifts in U.S. agriculture policy and practice would be required if Americans changed current consumption patterns to meet dietary guidelines.

Policies related to nutrition programs such as WIC and the Supplemental Nutrition Assistance Program (SNAP, also known as food stamps) could encourage participants to buy fruits and vegetables by allowing individuals to purchase items from local farmer's markets with their benefit dollars. This type of program has been executed in New York City and has demonstrated success thus far in increasing the amount of fruits and vegetables purchased via benefit dollars (The Council of the City of New York, 2011). School districts could allow the school lunch and breakfast program to purchase directly from local farmer's markets, and reimbursement rates could be higher for schools that purchase fresh fruits and vegetables.

Menu Labeling

Requiring restaurants and food vendors to provide clear and comprehensible nutrition information at the point of purchase has also been proposed (and passed as a national requirement in the 2010 health care reform bill). Consumers are often unaware of the nutritional content of the foods they eat, particularly the foods they eat outside the home where nutrition information is not readily available. Even nutrition professionals underestimate caloric content of restaurant meals (Backstrand, Wootan, Young, & Hurley, 1997), and the general public fares worse at guessing how many calories they are consuming when eating out (Young & Nestle, 1995). In one study, participants underestimated the caloric content of menu items by an average of 642 calories for unhealthy items and 43 calories for healthy items (Burton, Creyer, Keyes, & Huggins, 2006). Only 54% of the 287 largest chain restaurants in the United States provide any nutrition information to consumers, and of those, 86% provided this information via Web site, not in the restaurant (Wootan & Osborn, 2006). Nutrition information should be provided at the point of purchase (i.e., on the menu), where it can readily be factored in to the consumers' decisions. School cafeterias could also be required to provide nutrition information at the point of purchase for breakfast and lunch programs.

There is some scientific support for the potential effectiveness of menu labeling. Studies have shown that providing clear nutrition information on posters or labels at the point of purchase can reduce purchase of sugar-sweetened soft drinks from vending machines (Bergen & Yeh, 2006), increase purchase of healthy foods in college cafeterias (Buscher, Martin & Crocker, 2001), decrease the intent to purchase unhealthy menu items in a restaurant setting (Burton, Creyer, Kees, & Huggins, 2006), and decrease calories eaten. One study reported that parents would purchase approximately 100 fewer calories for their children from menus with nutrition labels, compared with menus without labels (Tandon, Wright, Zhou, Rogers, & Christakis, 2010). However, the research is not consistent. Other studies have shown no effect of menu labeling on the number of calories purchased (Elbel, Gyamfi, & Kersh, 2011; Elbel, Kersh, Brescoll, & Dixon, 2009; Finkelstein, Strombotne, Chan, & Krieger, 2011).

More than 80% of consumers report using nutrition labels at least "sometimes" when deciding what foods to purchase or eat (Borra, 2006). Even if only a small proportion of people actually utilize nutrition information when eating outside their home, this policy could have a big impact. One study estimated that even if only 10% of consumers made a 100 lower-calorie choice as a consequence of menu labeling (reducing intake by 100 calories), it would negate 41% of the 6.75 million pounds the U.S. population gains each year (Kuo, Jarosz, Simon, & Fielding, 2009). An additional benefit of a "menu labeling" policy may be that restaurants and vendors will reformulate their products to be healthier, or they may add healthy items to their menus. This was evident in processed foods after the Nutrition Labeling and Education Act was signed into law in 1990 (Variyam, 2005).

Barriers to Menu Labeling

There are some barriers to this approach as well. The restaurants and food vendors will incur the cost of creating new menu boards, and determining the caloric content of their food. This direct cost would be relatively minimal, approximately $220 per menu item or a one-time cost of $18,000 for a chain with 80 items (Wootan & Osborn, 2006). However, any cost is sure to inspire some strong opposition from the food industry. This happened in New York City, where the Department of Health passed a rule mandating nutrition information be placed on menu boards for chain restaurants. The restaurant industry successfully sued the Department of Health. However, now that menu labeling has been made federal law, there does not seem to be any escaping it, even through lawsuits.

One potential caveat is that merely providing nutrition information on menu boards may be insufficient to change behavior; additional consumer education instructing people on how to read labels and incorporate that information in order to make healthier choices may be necessary (Finkelstein, French, Variyam, & Haines, 2004). Many people don't know what to make of the "650 cal" labels next to the menu items without further education. Is it 650 out of 3,000? 50,000? Without knowing how many calories we should eat in a day, a label on a menu is meaningless. In point of fact, an evaluation of the New York City menu labeling initiative among low-income populations found no effect (Elbel et al., 2009), so it may be that among certain disadvantaged groups, menu labeling is meaningless without some sort of additional education putting those labels in context. One study reported that menu labels with additional info about the recommended daily caloric intake resulted in fewer calories eaten, whereas those with just the calorie labels for individual menu items did not (Roberto, Larsen, Agnew, Baik, & Brownell, 2010).

Advertising Restrictions

Regulation of media messages targeted to children and adolescents has been suggested as a means of tackling the obesity epidemic. Several other countries have implemented such a policy.

Each year, U.S. children see about 40,000 ads promoting snack foods and beverages, most of which are unhealthy (Institute of Medicine, 2005; Kaiser Family Foundation, 2004). Racial and ethnic minority groups are targeted disproportionately: African American children and teens see at least 50% more fast-food ads on TV than Caucasian children (Rudd Center for Food Policy and Obesity, 2010). Forty percent of parents say their child asks to go to McDonald's at least once a week, and 15% of preschoolers ask to go every day (Rudd Center for Food Policy and Obesity, 2010)! Although studies have yet to be conducted demonstrating the effectiveness of regulating media messages to children related to unhealthy foods, these types of interventions have been successful in other health outcomes such as tobacco control, and are a critical area for future research. One group of researchers estimated that a ban on fast-food advertising to children and adolescents would reduce the number of overweight children aged 3 to 11 years by 18% and the number of overweight adolescents (aged 12–18 years) by 14% (Chou, Rashad, & Grossman, 2006).

Ads qualify as business expenses and can be deducted to reduce taxable income for food companies. Policies aimed at eliminating this deduction would increase the price of advertising, and reduce the number of ads seen by children and adolescents by 33% to 40% (Chou et al., 2006). Further, it is estimated that eliminating the tax deductibility of fast-food advertising would produce declines in overweight prevalence of 5% and 7% for children and teens (Chou et al., 2006). Another study reported that banning food advertising to children under 12 years of age would decrease the average BMI by 0.38 kg/m^2 and lower the prevalence of obesity from 17.8% to 15.2% for boys and from 15.9% to 13.5% for girls (Veerman, Van Beeck, Barendregt, & Mackenbach, 2009).

Quebec, Sweden, Norway, and Finland have banned food advertising to children. In Sweden, no ads directed at children under 12 years of age are permitted. Such restrictions would certainly be challenged in court in the unlikely event that they were passed in the United States. Although restrictions on tobacco advertising to children have often held up under legal scrutiny, it is an open question whether restrictions on food advertisements would withstand similar lawsuits. Some food companies have voluntarily reduced advertising to children. You might think this is a good thing, but many times, companies voluntarily impose their own self-regulations in order to fend off stronger federal regulations. They essentially try to preemptively beat the government to the punch, hoping that if they impose their own limited restrictions, the government will give up on pursuing stricter standards. So it is unclear what, if any, effect these voluntary efforts will have.

Other efforts have been made to ban incentivizing poor food choices to children, such as offering toys in McDonald's Happy Meals. With the support of the Center for Science in the Public Interest (CSPI), a class action lawsuit was recently filed against McDonald's for baiting children into eating non-nutritious foods. This actually comes on the heels of the San Francisco Board of Supervisors passing an ordinance that toys can only be sold with foods meeting certain nutritional standards, which appears to be a direct hit on McDonald's battleship. The CSPI has previously been successful in advocating for lower levels of trans-fat in KFC products and modifying regulations for Kellogg cereal advertisements.

School Wellness Policies

The Child Nutrition and WIC Reauthorization Act requires all local education agencies that participate in the National School Lunch and Breakfast Programs to have a school wellness policy. These policies are required to cover the following areas: (1) goals for nutrition education, physical activity, and other school-based activities; (2) nutrition guidelines for foods served in schools (which cannot be less restrictive than the federal guidelines for reimbursable school meals); (3) a plan for measuring how well the policy is implemented; and (4) the involvement of parents, students, and school representatives in developing the policy (Story et al., 2009). Other than these broad-stroke guidelines, school districts have virtually complete leeway in designing their own policies. This is good in that it allows schools in Baltimore City to design a different policy than schools in rural Nebraska. However, it also means that there is a huge variety of policies, and that some of them are pretty shoddy.

Barriers to Successful Prevention Policies

The state of the economy is an important factor in determining whether a particular intervention is feasible. In times of state and federal budget shortfalls, public health policies and interventions are less likely to be funded than when there are budget surpluses. Therefore, any new policies or programs must find sustainable funding through either increasing various taxes or making budget cuts to other federal investments. These options are not very popular, politically, especially for prevention policies that actually take considerable time to demonstrate positive outcomes on society. It is much easier to just maintain the status quo. Thus, without a groundswell of social and political will, it is not likely that we'll see obesity prevention policies such as junk food taxes enacted at the federal level any time soon. (Menu labeling appears to be an exception, as it was tucked into the health care reform bill without many people noticing). Another barrier is that most people still think that what we eat (and therefore, what we weigh) is a matter of personal responsibility and choice, not a consequence of our environments. So there is not (yet) a ton of support for policy interventions, particularly those that cost money.

Finally, as described with other types of prevention efforts above, single policies are unlikely to be effective given the complex and multilevel web of causal pathways leading to obesity. A combination of approaches targeting multiple levels of influence will likely be required to have an impact on obesity rates.

CONTROVERSIES

There are several areas of disagreement, or areas in desperate need of more research, when it comes to obesity prevention.

Voluntary vs. Mandated

Given the barriers to passing various policies or implementing obesity prevention programs, relying on voluntary efforts by the food industry is not an uncommon solution. We mentioned how at times, these voluntary efforts are really just lip-service to ward off stronger regulations or laws. However, there are other times when public–private partnerships can be beneficial. For example, the largest soda companies in the United States voluntarily pulled sugary sodas from schools by 2009. Although they may have had ulterior motives, this move is surely beneficial. Another recent partnership has emerged between Wal-Mart and Michelle Obama. Wal-Mart announced that it would make thousands of its packaged foods lower in salt, fat, and sugar, as well as reduce the price of fruits and vegetables (Stolberg, 2011). These plans came out of discussions with Michelle Obama, who has spearheaded many initiatives related to obesity prevention.

There are some people who believe that partnerships with industry are akin to selling your soul to the devil. There are others who believe that these partnerships are realistically the only way to accomplish anything, even if the end result is sub-optimal. There's no right answer. Relying on industry to self-regulate may, at times, be the only way to make any sort of progress towards obesity prevention, even if this progress is far less than ideal. Other times, this strategy is tantamount to letting the wolves guard the hen house.

Cost Effectiveness

You might have noticed that there are not many studies documenting the effectiveness of different obesity prevention programs. Of the research that has been done looking at effectiveness, there is not much out there in the way of showing that various programs are cost effective. If a program works, but costs $20,000 per person to implement, it does not have a very good chance of being adopted. In order to get decision makers to buy into obesity prevention programs, whether in a public or private setting, it would be extremely helpful to have more information about which interventions are likely to get the most bang for our buck. This is especially important in a world of limited resources, where we typically have to decide between programs X, Y, and Z. Since we can't do it all, we have to decide which program represents the best investment. Cost-effectiveness research can also help build (or destroy) a case for action. If advocacy organizations can point to research stating that improving school lunches will save taxpayers $10 million because fewer children will become obese, and fewer will develop diabetes, and there will be lower associated health care costs—then that provides a much stronger argument than "because it's the right thing to do," or "we think it will work," or "pretty pretty please, with sprinkles on top?"

One Step at a Time?

We have mentioned no less than three dozen times (at least it feels that way) how individual strategies are not likely to work in isolation. This may seem somewhat discouraging, since the likelihood that state or federal governments will pass bills including comprehensive school food reform, *and* school physical activity standards, *and* junk food taxes, *and* agriculture policy changes, *and* advertising restrictions to children is pretty much nil. So where does that leave us? Well, no one said that obesity prevention interventions have to be undertaken all at once. What we said was that if we are looking for an effect on obesity rates, we aren't likely to see anything if we are looking only at one program at a time on its own. Thus, there is a danger in evaluating obesity prevention programs in isolation and concluding that they don't work. They may work, but only when piggybacking on several other programs and policies working in tandem. In terms of implementing obesity prevention interventions, one step at a time may be the only way to go, provided that the lack of immediate results doesn't force decision makers to pull the plug prematurely. We simply need to be cautious in interpreting the research evaluating the outcomes of these interventions.

Evaluations that look at multilevel, multicomponent prevention strategies are difficult but necessary. One such evaluation, Shape up Somerville, has demonstrated very encouraging results (Economos et al., 2007). This program involved changing school food, creating a health-based curriculum both during and after school, changing the school environment, using parent and community outreach, working with local restaurants to increase healthy options, providing safe routes to walk or bike to school, and conducting weight assessments in schools. Children in the community receiving the intervention had lower BMI z-scores than children in two communities who did not receive the intervention. So although we have been quick to point to the difficulties associated with treating and preventing obesity, please know that there is hope, and it can be done. In fact, more of it needs to be done and rigorously evaluated.

SUMMARY

We have described some of the more popular prevention strategies that have been proposed or attempted, though there are dozens (if not hundreds) of other options. Communities, governments, schools, industries, workplaces, organizations, and even countries are interested in obesity prevention at an increasing rate. According to the Trust for America's Health (2011) annual report on obesity-related policies in the United States, obesity prevention policies have become much more

TABLE 6.1 **OBESITY PREVENTION POLICIES IN U.S. STATES, 2005 AND 2010**

Policy	2005	2010
Strong nutrition standards for school meals	4 states	20 states and DC
Nutritional standards for competitive foods sold in schools	6 states	28 states and DC
BMI screening or weight assessments in schools	4 states	20 states
Programs linking farms to schools	1 state	23 states and DC
Sales tax on soda or snacks	17 states	33 states
Menu labeling (prior to federal menu labeling legislation)	0	5 states
Legislation to ensure "complete streets" (i.e., streets that are safe for pedestrians, bicyclists, motorists, and transit users)	0	13 states

From Trust for America's Health, 2011.

popular over the past five years (see Table 6.1). A greater number of states have enacted various prevention policies by 2010 compared with 2005. This is encouraging, but more work needs to be done demonstrating that these policies actually work, and at what cost.

NOTES

[1] In reality, recidivism rates for prisoners are over 67%, which is not so great either.
[2] You can see the ads here: http://www.nyc.gov/html/doh/html/cdp/cdp_pan_pop.shtml

REFERENCES

Anderson, L. M., Quinn, T. A., Glanz, K., Ramirez, G., Kahwati, L. C., Johnson, D. B., . . . Katz, D. L. (2009). The effectiveness of worksite nutrition and physical activity interventions for controlling employee overweight and obesity: A systematic review. *American Journal of Preventive Medicine, 37*(4), 340–357.

Anderson, S. E., & Whitaker, R. C. (2009). Prevalence of obesity among US preschool children in different racial and ethnic groups. *Archives of Pediatric and Adolescent Medicine, 163*(4), 344–348.

Andreyeva, T., Chaloupka, F. J., & Brownell, K. D. (2011). Estimating the potential of taxes on sugar-sweetened beverages to reduce consumption and generate revenue. *Preventive Medicine, 52*(6), 413–416.

Ashe, M., Jernigan, D., Kline, R., & Galaz, R. (2003). Land use planning and the control of alcohol, tobacco, firearms, and fast food restaurants. *Journal of the American Public Health Association, 93,* 1404–1408.

Backstrand, J., Wootan, M. G., Young, L. R., & Hurley, J. (1997). *Fat chance.* Washington, DC: Center for Science in the Public Interest.

Benson, L., Baer, H. J., & Kaelber, D. C. (2009). Trends in the diagnosis of overweight and obesity in children and adolescents: 1999–2007. *Pediatrics, 123,* e153–e158.

Bergen, D., & Yeh, M. C. (2006). Effects of energy-content labels and motivational posters on sales of sugar-sweetened beverages: Stimulating sales of diet drinks among adults study. *Journal of the American Dietetic Association, 106,* 1866–1869.

Bluford, D. A. A., Sherry, B., & Scanlon, K. S. (2007). Interventions to prevent or treat obesity in preschool children: A review of evaluated programs. *Obesity, 15,* 1356–1372.

Booth, K. M., Pinkston, M. M., & Poston, W. S. C. (2005). Obesity and the built environment. *Journal of the American Dietetic Association, 105,* S110–S117.

Borra, S. (2006). Consumer perspectives on food labels. *American Journal of Clinical Nutrition, 83*(Suppl.), 1235S.

Brown, T., Avenell, A., Edmunds, L. D., Moore, H., Whittaker, V., Avery, L., Summerbell, C. (2009). Systematic review of long-term lifestyle interventions to prevent weight gain and morbidity in adults. *Obesity Reviews, 10*(6), 627–638.

Brown, T., & Summerbell, C. (2009). Systematic review of school-based interventions that focus on changing dietary intake and physical activity levels to prevent childhood obesity: An update to the obesity guidance produced by the National Institute for Health and Clinical Excellence. *Obesity Reviews, 10,* 110–141.

Burton, S., Creyer, E. H., Kees, J., & Huggins, K. (2006). Attacking the obesity epidemic: The potential health benefits of providing nutritional information in restaurants. *American Journal of Public Health, 96,* 1669–1675.

Buscher, L. A., Martin, K. A., & Crocker, S. (2001). Point-of-purchase messages framed in terms of cost, convenience, taste, and energy improve healthful snack selection in a college foodservice setting. *Journal of the American Dietetic Association, 101,* 909–913.

Chou, S. Y., Rashad, I., & Grossman, M. (2006). *Fast-food restaurant advertising on television and its influence on childhood obesity.* National Bureau of Economic Research Working Paper No. 11879. Retrieved from www.nber.org/papers/w11879

Community Preventive Services. (2010). *Obesity prevention and control: Provider-oriented interventions.* Retrieved February 6, 2011, from http://www.thecommunityguide.org/obesity/provider.html

The Council of the City of New York. (2011). *Food stamp use at greenmarkets doubles in 2010.* Retrieved April 18, 2011, from http://council.nyc.gov/html/releases/greenmarket_ebt_doubles_01_03_11.shtml

Davison, K. K., Werder, J. L., & Lawson, C. T. (2008). Children's active commuting to school: Current knowledge and future directions. *Preventing Chronic Disease, 5*(3), 1–11.

Dobbins, M., De Corby, K., Robeson, P., Husson, H., & Tirillis, D. (2009). School-based physical activity programs for promoting physical activity and fitness in children and adolescents aged 6–18. *Cochrane Database Systematic Reviews,* Jan 21;(1):CD007651.

Dorsey, R. R., Eberhardt, M. S., & Ogden, C. L. (2009). Racial/ethnic differences in weight perception. *Obesity, 17*(4), 790–795.

Economos, C. D., Hyatt, R. R., Goldberg, J. P., Must, A., Naumova, E. N., Collins, J. J., Nelson, M. E. (2007). A community intervention reduces BMI z-score in children: Shape Up Somerville first year results. *Obesity, 15,* 1325–1336.

Elbel, B., Gyamfi, J., & Kersh, R. (2011). Child and adolescent fast-food choice and the influence of calorie labeling: A natural experiment. *International Journal of Obesity, 35*(4), 493–500.

Elbel, B., Kersh, R., Brescoll, V. L., & Dixon, L. B. (2009). Calorie labeling and food choices: A first look at the effects on low-income people in New York City. *Health Affairs, 28,* 1110–1121.

Epstein, L. H., Dearing, K. K., Roba, L. G., & Finkelstein, E. (2010). The influence of taxes and subsidies on energy purchased in an experimental purchasing study. *Psychological Science, 21*(3), 406–414.

Epstein, L. H., Handley, E. A., Dearing, K. K., Cho, D. D., Roemmich, J. N., Paluch, R. A.,...Spring, B. (2006). Purchases of food in youth: Influence of price and income. *Psychological Science, 17,* 82–89.

Finkelstein, E., French, S., Variyam, J. N., & Haines, P. S. (2004). Pros and cons of proposed interventions to promote healthy eating. *American Journal of Preventive Medicine, 27,* 163–171.

Finkelstein, E. A., Strombotne, K. L., Chan, N. L., & Krieger, J. (2011). Mandatory menu labeling in one fast-food chain in King County, Washington. *American Journal of Preventive Medicine, 40*(2), 122–127.

French, S. A. (2003). Pricing effects on food choices. *Journal of Nutrition, 133,* 841S–843S.

Glanz, K., Basil, M., Mailbach, E., Goldberg, J., & Snyder, D. (1998). Why Americans eat what they do: Taste, nutrition, cost, convenience and weight control concerns as influences on food consumption. *Journal of the American Dietetic Association, 98,* 1118–1126.

Gordon, R., McDermott, L., Stead, M., & Angus, K. (2006). The effectiveness of social marketing interventions for health improvement: What's the evidence? *Public Health, 120*(12), 1133–1139.

Gostin, L. O. (2007). Law as a tool to facilitate healthier lifestyles and prevent obesity. *Journal of the American Medical Association, 287,* 87–90.

Harris, K. C., Kuramoto, L. K., Schulzer, M., & Retallack, J. E. (2009). Effect of school-based physical activity interventions on body mass index in children: A meta-analysis. *Canadian Medical Association Journal, 180*(7), 719–726.

Harper, A., Shattuck, A., Holt-Gimenez, E., Alkon, A., & Lambrick, F. (2009). *Food policy councils: Lessons learned.* Institute for Food and Development Policy. Retrieved from http://foodsecurity.org/pub/Food_Policy_Councils_Report.pdf

Horgen, K. B., & Brownell, K. D. (2002). Comparison of price change and health message interventions in promoting healthy food choices. *Health Psychology, 21*(5), 505–512.

Institute of Medicine. (2005). *Preventing childhood obesity: Health in the balance.* Washington, DC: National Academies Press.

Jacobson, M. F., & Brownell, K. D. (2000). Small taxes on soft drinks and snack foods to promote health. *American Journal of Public Health, 90,* 854–857.

Justus, M. B., Ryan, K. W., Rockenbach, J., Katterapalli, C., & Card-Higginson, P. (2007). Lessons learned while implementing a legislated school policy: Body mass index assessments among Arkansas's public school students. *Journal of School Health, 77*(10), 706–713.

Kaiser Family Foundation. (2004). *The role of media in childhood obesity.* Menlo Park, CA: Henry J. Kaiser Family Foundation. Retrieved from http://www.kff.org/entmedia/entmedia022404pkg.cfm

Katz, D. L., O'Connell, M., Njike, V. Y., Yeh, M. C., & Nawaz, H. (2008). Strategies for the prevention and control of obesity in the school setting: Systematic review and meta-analysis. *International Journal of Obesity, 32*(12), 1780–1789.

Kubik, M. Y., Story, M., & Rieland, G. (2007). Developing school-based BMI screening and parent notification programs: Findings from focus groups with parents of elementary school students. *Health Education & Behavior, 34*(4), 622–633.

Kuchler, F., Tegene, A., & Harris, J. M. (2004). *Taxing snack foods: What to expect for diet and tax revenues.* Current Issues in Economics of Food Markets. Agriculture Information Bulletin No. 747-08.

Kuo, T., Jarosz, C. J., Simon, P., & Fielding, J. E. (2009). Menu labeling as a potential strategy for combating the obesity epidemic: A health impact assessment. *American Journal of Public Health, 99*(9), 1680–1686.

Kweon, B. S., Shin, W. H., Folzenlogen, R., & Kim, J. H. (2007). *Children and transportation: Identifying environments that foster walking and biking to school.* College Station, TX: Southwest Region University Transportation Center and the Texas Transportation Institute.

Lee, S. M., Burgeson, C. R., Fulton, J. E., & Spain, C. G. (2007). Physical education and physical activity: Results from the School Health Policies and Programs Study 2006. *Journal of School Health, 77*(8), 435–463.

Lemmens, V. E., Oenema, A., Klepp, K. I., Henriksen, H. B., & Brug, J. (2008). A systematic review of the evidence regarding efficacy of obesity prevention interventions among adults. *Obesity Reviews*, 9(5), 446–455.

Louthan, M. V., Lafferty-Oza, M. J., Smith, E. R., Hornang, C. A., Franco, S., & Theriot, J. A. (2005). Diagnosis and treatment frequency of overweight children and adolescents at well child visits. *Clinical Pediatrics*, 44, 57–61.

Nihiser, A. J., Lee, S. M., Wechsler, H., McKenna, M., Odom, E., Reinold, C., ... Grummer-Strawn, L. (2007). Body mass index measurement in schools. *Journal of School Health*, 77(10), 651–671.

O'Toole, T. P., Anderson, S., Miller, C., & Guthrie, J. (2007). Nutrition services and foods and beverages available at school: Results from the School Health Policies and Programs Study 2006. *Journal of School Health*, 77(8), 500–521.

Raczynski, J. M., Thompson, J. W., Phillips, M. M., Ryan, K. W., & Cleveland, H. W. (2009). Arkansas Act 1220 of 2003 to reduce childhood obesity: Its implementation and impact on child and adolescent body mass index. *Journal of Public Health Policy*, 30, S124–S140.

Roberto, C. A., Larsen, P. D., Agnew, H., Baik, J., & Brownell, K. D. (2010). Evaluating the impact of menu labeling on food choices and intake. *American Journal of Public Health*, 21, 312–318.

Rudd Center for Food Policy and Obesity. (2010). *Fast food FACTS: Evaluating fast food nutrition and marketing to youth*. Retrieved February 16, 2011, from http://www.fastfoodmarketing.org/

Saunders, K. L. (2007). Preventing obesity in pre-school children: A literature review. *Journal of Public Health*, 29(4), 368–375.

Smith, T. A., Lin, B. H., & Lee, J. Y. (2010). *Taxing caloric sweetened beverages: Potential effects on beverage consumption, calorie intake, and obesity*. Economic Research Report 100, U.S. Department of Agriculture, Economic Research Service, July 2010.

Snelling, A. M., Korba, C., & Burkey, A. (2007). The National School Lunch and competitive food offerings and purchasing behaviors of high school students. *Journal of School Health*, 77(10), 701–705.

Soler, R. E., Leeks, K. D., Buchanan, L. R., Brownson, R. C., Heath, G. W., & Task Force on Community Preventive Services. (2010). Point-of-decision prompts to increase stair use: A systematic review update. *American Journal of Preventive Medicine, 2*(Suppl. 1), S292–S300.

Stolberg, S. G. (2011, January 20). Wal-Mart shifts strategy to promote healthy foods. *New York Times.* Retrieved February 16, 2011, from http://www.nytimes.com/2011/01/20/business/20walmart.html

Story, M., Kaphingst, K. M., Robinson-O'Brien, R., & Glanz, K. (2008). Creating healthy food and eating environments: Policy and environmental approaches. *Annual Review of Public Health, 29,* 253–272.

Story, M., Nanney, M. S., & Schwartz, M. B. (2009). Schools and obesity prevention: Creating school environments and policies to promote healthy eating and physical activity. *Milbank Quarterly, 87,* 71–100.

Summerbell, C. D., Waters, E., Edmunds, L. D., Kelly, S., Brown, T., & Campbell, K. J. (2005). Interventions for preventing obesity in children. *Cochrane Database Systematic Reviews,* Jul 20 (3), CD001871.

Tandon, P. S., Wright, J., Zhou, C., Rogers, C. B., & Christakis, D. A. (2010). Nutrition menu labeling may lead to lower-calorie restaurant meal choices for children. *Pediatrics, 125,* 244–248.

Task Force on Community Preventive Services. (2009). A recommendation to improve employee weight status through worksite health promotion programs targeting nutrition, physical activity, or both. *American Journal of Preventive Medicine, 37*(4), 358–359.

The Nielsen Company. (2011). *Average TV viewing per day.* Retrieved February 6, 2011, from http://blog.nielsen.com/nielsenwire/wp-content/uploads/2009/11/avg_tv_viewing.png

Trudeau, F., & Shephard, R. J. (2008). Physical education, school physical activity, school sports and academic performance. *International Journal of Behavioral Nutrition and Physical Activity, 5,* 10.

Trust for America's Health. (2011). *F as in fat: How obesity threatens America's future, 2010.* Retrieved from http://healthyamericans.org/reports/obesity2010/

U.S. Preventive Services Task Force. (2003). *Screening for obesity in adults: Recommendations and rationale.* Retrieved February 5, 2011, from http://www.uspreventiveservicestaskforce.org/3rduspstf/obesity/obesrr.htm

U.S. Preventive Services Task Force. (2010). Screening for obesity in children and adolescents: US Preventive Services Task Force recommendation statement. *Pediatrics, 125,* 361–367.

Variyam, J. N. (2005). *Nutrition labeling in the food-away-from-home sector: An economic assessment.* Economic Research Report Number 4. Washington, DC: United States Department of Agriculture Economic Research Service.

Veerman, J. L., Van Beeck, E. F., Barendregt, J. J., & Mackenbach, J. P. (2009). By how much would limiting TV food advertising reduce childhood obesity. *European Journal of Public Health, 19*(4), 365–369.

Wilson, A. R., & McAlpine, D. D. (2006). The effectiveness of screening for obesity in primary care: Weighing the evidence. *Medical Care Research and Review, 63,* 570–598.

Wootan, M. G., & Osborn, M. (2006). Availability of nutrition information from chain restaurants in the United States. *American Journal of Preventive Medicine, 30*(3), 266–268.

Young, L. R., & Nestle, M. (1995). Portion sizes in dietary assessment: Issues and policy implications. *Nutrition Reviews, 53,* 149–158.

Conclusion: Global and Future Trends

IN CASE YOU SKIPPED TO THE END...

We have spent the previous hundreds of pages telling you everything you need to know about obesity. In case you are one of those people who prefer the bottom line, here is the abridged version (although be assured—you're missing out).

What Is Obesity?

We started by describing how overweight and obesity are defined or measured, most commonly with the body mass index (BMI of 25 to 29 kg/m² = *overweight*; 30 kg/m² or higher = *obese*; 40 kg/m² or higher = *extreme obesity*), which is derived from a formula using height and weight only. Perhaps, to no surprise, we now know there are many flaws with using BMI, and one of the most contested aspects is that it does not distinguish between muscle mass and fat mass. So, you can have an NFL running back with 8% body fat and a BMI of 35 kg/m², whereas someone watching the game from the stands eating nachos and hot dogs can have 30% body fat with a BMI of 26 kg/m². Obviously, it is best to measure body fat directly, since that is what we are really interested in. However, this is costly, in terms of both time and money. So until researchers start getting paid like NBA stars (we will continue dreaming), it is unlikely that we'll see studies discontinue using BMI in favor of percent body fat by DEXA scan. If you plan on following a career in obesity research, you will see how much easier it is to collect BMI data, but you would be wise to include some other measures of obesity in your studies, such as waist circumference, waist-to-hip ratio, or body composition (if you can afford it). Hopefully, someone will invent some cheap and easy way to measure body fat directly, but we're not holding our breath.

Why We Care About Obesity

Obesity is bad for our health. People who are obese are more likely to suffer from a variety of negative health consequences—medical, psychological, and social in nature. Some of the not-so-great things associated with obesity include high blood pressure, high cholesterol, type 2 diabetes, cardiovascular disease, stroke, musculoskeletal problems, sleep apnea, several types of cancer, depression, anxiety, reduced quality of life, lower academic performance, decreased job outlook, social stigma, dementia, reduced life expectancy, and mortality (for references, see Chapters 3 and 4). We could go on and on, but this is supposed to be a concise summary.

Now, we might not be as concerned about these associations if only 1% of the population were obese. The problem is, one in three Americans is obese, and another one in three is overweight. Any math whiz has already realized that the majority of Americans, therefore, do not fall within a healthy weight range. In recent years, this "epidemic" has increasingly affected children and adolescents, with nearly one in three children and adolescents in the United States clinically overweight or obese; and these figures are higher among certain racial and ethnic subpopulations, or low-income groups. Unfortunately, despite our increased knowledge and research on obesity, these rates have increased drastically over the past several decades across the globe, and the trend shows no sign of abating.

This growing pandemic means that the negative health effects of obesity are becoming more and more common; we are seeing greater morbidity and mortality and greater associated costs. As an example, about one third of cancer cases in the United States, 340,000 cases, could be prevented each year if Americans had healthier diets, exercised regularly, and limited alcohol intake (World Cancer Research Fund International, 2011). In large part, because of the pervasiveness of obesity, poor diet, and inactivity, cancer will kill more than 13.2 million people worldwide each year by 2030; twice the number killed in 2008 (International Agency for Research on Cancer, 2011).

The United States and other high-income nations have managed to suppress some of the damage that obesity can cause on a population level, as we have access to medication for high cholesterol and diabetes. So the consequences of obesity are not as severe as they could be, although this still wreaks havoc on our health care system. Unfortunately, in many other countries across the globe, access to medical care is limited. The effects of obesity will be felt to a much greater degree in these nations.

Why Has Obesity Increased Over Time?

To answer this question, we must ask what causes obesity; specifically:

1. What causes a specific individual person to become obese?
2. What causes a large proportion of the American (or any other country; more on that in a bit) population to become (and stay) obese?

In both cases, the *simple* answer is caloric imbalance. Too many calories taken in and not enough expended. But what causes this caloric imbalance? At the individual level, it is a combination of a person's genes and environment. On an individual level, genes are hugely important in determining why one person is obese, whereas his neighbor is stick-thin. Other factors are still critically important, however, such as how those two individuals were raised, the weights and behaviors of their parents, whether they were breastfed, how much television (TV) they watch, the communities and environments they live in, and so on.

In regards to the second question, why is one third of our population now obese when this was not the case 30 years ago? To paraphrase Bill Clinton, "It's the environment, stupid." Our gene pool hasn't changed much in the past 10,000 years, let alone the past 30. What has changed is how we live. We are less active now that we have cars, TVs, computers, Segways, escalators, and elevators. We eat more now that we have super cheap, convenient, and highly accessible food that we no longer have to hunt and gather ourselves, and in fact are marketed for us to eat when we aren't even hungry. Of course, there are literally hundreds of different factors that contribute to the increase in calories consumed and the decrease in calories expended. Everything from school lunches to soda advertisements to the distance to the nearest park has been implicated in raising the risk of obesity.

One controversy that receives a lot of attention is whether to blame poorer diet or lower activity level for societal increases in obesity. To be sure, the answer to this question is more complex than picking one over the other. With that said, although the McDonald's and Coca-Colas of the world would have you believe that physical activity is more critical (because that exempts them from responsibility), diet bears more responsibility for obesity at the individual and societal level. Physical activity is wonderful, and we should all be doing more of it for a variety of reasons; but when it comes to our weights, what we eat individually and as a population is simply more important when considering how we got to this point and how we can reverse the trend.

OBESITY ACROSS THE GLOBE

We have spent most of the book talking about the state of affairs in the United States. Unfortunately, the United States is not the only place that has seen rising rates of obesity over time. The prevalence of obesity across the globe doubled between 1980 and 2008 (Finucane et al., 2011). Similar to the trends seen in the United States over the past several decades, obesity has been rising in many other countries across the globe. Many countries appear to be catching up rather quickly to the United States in regards to overall obesity prevalence. In fact, obesity is increasing in some countries two to five times as fast as we saw in the United States (Popkin & Gordon-Larsen, 2004). Figure 7.1 illustrates how the mean BMI has increased over the past 30 years in several countries across the globe.

It is estimated that approximately 1.5 billion adults are currently overweight across the world, and another 500 million are obese (World Health Organization, 2011). Approximately 150 million children are overweight, and 50 million are obese (International Obesity Task Force, 2011). The number of obese people across the globe now dwarfs the 850 million who are underweight (Runge, 2007). If we continue on our current path, by 2015, 2.3 billion adults will be overweight and 700 million will be obese (World Health Organization, 2011). Largely because of obesity, the deaths due to diabetes worldwide are projected to increase by more than 50% over the next 10 years (World Health Organization, 2011).

You can see the 25 countries with the highest obesity rates in Figure 7.2. Of note, the United States is ninth. Nauru, a tiny island in the Pacific Ocean, actually has the highest prevalence

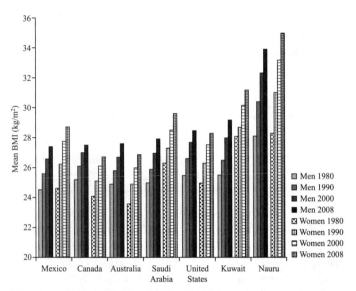

FIGURE 7.1 Mean BMI from 1980 to 2008 in several countries. From Finucane et al., 2011.

of obesity, with about three in four adults qualifying as obese, and between 93% and 97% of adults falling in the category of overweight or obese. To give some perspective, if you worked in an office of 40 people in Nauru, only two of them would fall in a normal weight category. In Nauru and many other remote Pacific islands, obesity rates have exploded in recent years. The story of Nauru highlights the nature versus nurture debate that we discussed in Chapter 2.

In the first half of the 20th century, the residents of Nauru used to exclusively grow and procure their own food, as the island was pretty far removed from modern society. This meant a very healthy diet of seafood and locally grown produce, with minimal added fat or sugar. It also meant that residents expended a great deal of energy growing and preparing meals, requiring high activity levels. During that time period, Pacific Islanders were reported to have relatively muscular physiques, though obesity was associated with a high social position

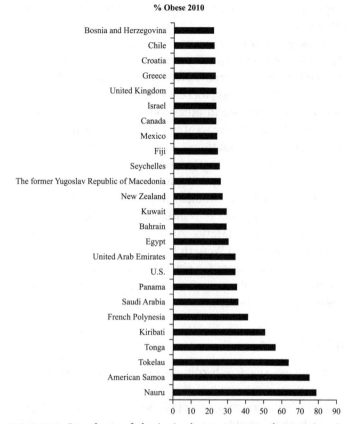

FIGURE 7.2 Prevalence of obesity in the top 25 most obese nations in the world, 2010. From World Health Organization, 2011.

(Hodge, Dowse, & Zimmet, 1996) as those with a higher status did not have to expend physical energy to grow and cook food, and had greater access to food. Then, in the 1960s, someone discovered that Nauru was incredibly rich in phosphate. Very quickly, companies seeking this natural resource descended on Nauru by plane and boat. Practically overnight, Nauru went from having virtually no access to anything other than locally grown fruits and vegetables and seafood to being inundated with highly processed, energy dense, and generally unhealthy convenience foods. Of course, given the choice between grilled fish and fried chicken with a side of Coke (at a much cheaper price and greater level of convenience), islanders chose the latter. No longer having to expend energy to prepare their own foods, and shifting to Westernized diets of highly processed, high-fat foods, rates of obesity skyrocketed. Although obesity rates were high in Nauru relative to other countries even as far back as 1975 (which was a few years after the influx of processed convenience foods), they shot from 63% of men to more than 80% of men being obese by 1994 (Hodge et al., 1996). The average BMI went from approximately 28 kg/m^2 in 1980 to 34 and 35 kg/m^2 in 2008 for men and women, respectively (Finucane et al., 2011). Now, nearly half of Nauru islanders suffer from diabetes as a consequence (Marks, 2010). As is the case with Nauru, many have pointed to Western (read: American) lifestyle influences (e.g., a preference for sedentary activities and a preponderance of high-calorie convenience food) as a reason for the global spread of obesity.

A Double-Edged Sword

Although obesity has become a problem in many different countries across the globe, there are several differences in the pattern of who becomes obese (Monteiro, Conde, Lu, & Popkin, 2004). In the United States and other high-income nations, the poor and less educated are more likely to be obese than wealthier groups. In low- and middle-income countries, obesity first increases among the higher echelons of society, while the poor suffer from hunger and food insecurity. As countries become wealthier, the burden of obesity shifts to the poor (Popkin & Gordon-Larsen, 2004).

This has lead to a serious problem. On the one hand, the poor living in these less wealthy, developing nations are starving. On the other hand, the well-to-do are suffering from obesity and all of the related diseases associated with excess weight. This is a serious problem because programs to address undernutrition can increase obesity; and conversely, programs to address obesity can increase undernutrition. So what do you do in a country that faces the simultaneous health threats of obesity and undernutrition? Really, if you know the answer to this question, please contact us immediately. There are many people interested in the answer.

WHAT NOW?

Now that we can all agree that obesity is a problem, what can we do about it? Well, for the 500 million people worldwide who are already obese, treatment is the obvious answer.

Treating Obesity

There are several different categories of weight-loss treatment. These treatments often follow a progression from less intensive to more intensive. The first weight-loss attempts are typically self-initiated diets. These are the New Year's resolutions, the "I'm cutting out chocolate for Lent" diets, the people who start trying to run on the treadmill before work, and things such as the Atkins or South Beach diets. This category basically consists of anything you might find in the "Self Help" section of your local bookstore. Slightly more intensive are the programs such as Weight Watchers and Jenny Craig, as they may involve group meetings and structured programs.

Individuals may cycle through dozens of these diets before moving up to the next level: behavioral or lifestyle modification. This type of treatment includes modifying a person's diet, physical activity patterns, and other behaviors and cognitions related to weight and weight loss. These programs are often conducted under the supervision of a health professional, such as a psychologist or dietician, or both. Another direction that individuals often go after several failed self-initiated diets is taking over-the-counter weight loss pills, herbal treatments, or prescription medication from their physicians. Others may attempt following very-low-calorie diets under medical supervision. Finally, as a last resort, after all else has failed, we arrive at weight-loss surgery, which seems to be one of the only treatments that lead to significant, long-term, sustainable weight loss—unfortunately, this method also brings additional risks. See Chapter 6 for more.

How do all these treatments fare in terms of success rates? First, a word about "success." Most health professionals define successful weight loss to mean a sustained (i.e., at least two year) weight loss of 5% to 10% of initial body weight. So, for your typical 200-pound individual, he or she needs to lose 10 to 20 pounds and keep it off for two years. This amount of weight loss can be achieved through lifestyle or behavior modification programs or prescription medication (as long as you continue to take the medication for two years), although not without significant effort.

Ask an obese person what he or she would personally consider to be a successful weight loss, however, and you will get a very different answer. The average obese person seeking weight-loss treatment wants to lose 25% or more of body weight, and will not be satisfied with less. So, for that 200-pound person, you need to raise that 10- to 20-pound weight-loss goal to a 50-pound weight loss. Unfortunately, the only way to reliably achieve this kind of weight loss is through surgery. Of course, the rare person can catch lightning in a bottle and lose 100 pounds by eating only Subway sandwiches, applying to be on a weight-loss television show, or by enrolling in a lifestyle modification program. However, the *vast majority* of people return to their original weights by five years after weight-loss treatment. The average weight loss 4.5 years after treatment is 2.1% of initial body weight (Anderson, Konz, Frederich, & Wood, 2001). For our aforementioned 200-pound friend, that means a loss of only 4 pounds despite wanting to lose 50. Pretty depressing, right?

Preventing Obesity

Because success rates following obesity treatment are pretty horrendous, many people have said that we need to instead focus on preventing people from becoming obese in the first place. Generally, with prevention, you want to intervene before people actually become obese. Logically, it makes sense to target children. Since children spend so much time in school and because school environments have been linked to obesity, many prevention initiatives have been conducted in a school setting. These interventions typically involve a number of components, including improving school food, increasing physical activity, health and nutrition education, and BMI screening. Overall, school-based interventions have shown some limited success in some studies, and no effect in others. This has not discouraged most researchers, as new initiatives surface quite frequently.

As much as we'd like to quell the obesity epidemic among our nation's youth in one fell swoop, we can't just completely ignore adults, so there are a few different prevention programs that have been developed for the workplace. These programs may involve education, counseling, or changing workplace policies and environments. Additionally, health care providers can do BMI screening. Much like school-based interventions, there is some evidence that workplace obesity prevention programs can be successful, though many studies show no effect.

One problem with most of the prevention programs that have been studied is that they focus on the individual, when we know it is the environment that has led to the rapid increases in obesity prevalence across the United States and elsewhere. Some community and policy approaches have been proposed and tested in recent years. These interventions include:

● Changing the built environment to make it more conducive to physical activity (e.g., increasing "walkability," using smart growth policies, building bike paths, changing zoning codes).

283

- Changing the food environment to facilitate access to healthy foods (e.g., fresh food financing, social marketing, changes to zoning codes, healthy stores initiatives, community gardens).
- Creating food policy councils.
- Instating junk food taxes and subsidizing healthy foods.
- Restructuring agriculture policy to direct subsidies to fresh fruits and vegetables.
- Mandating that restaurants and vending machines provide nutrition information at the point of purchase.
- Restricting advertising and availability of unhealthy foods to children.
- Creating school wellness policies to improve the school environment.
- Forming partnerships with various companies and getting them to voluntarily change industry practices.

Most of these prevention strategies have not been evaluated at all, let alone with rigorous controlled studies. After all, it would be basically impossible to say "we're going to randomize half of the states to ban unhealthy food ads to kids, and the other half to continue with the status quo and see what happens." The other problem is that the prevalence of obesity shot up over time because of many different changes to our environments and economies, so we wouldn't necessarily expect that changing one feature of our environment or policy landscape would result in any measurable change in obesity rates. We will need to restructure many different factors simultaneously if we are going to see a noticeable reversal of the epidemic at all, let alone within the duration of a research study. Essentially, we need to work on making healthier choices the default option, instead of the unhealthy choice always being the easiest to make.

One encouraging sign is that obesity prevention is becoming more of a national priority. Michelle Obama recently announced her goal of ending childhood obesity within a generation with her "Let's Move" campaign.[1] This campaign seeks to change many different factors related to diet and physical activity, across many different settings. It calls for changes to our schools, homes, and communities. It enlists the help of parents, pediatricians, the food industry, and all levels of government. This type of high-visibility initiative has done wonders to put obesity prevention on the agenda for many individuals, communities, businesses, and organizations. Time will tell whether this campaign can inspire changes to effectively reduce childhood obesity levels.

Global Solutions

Preventing obesity is on the global agenda as well. The World Health Organization has put forth guidelines to address diet, activity, and obesity (World Health Organization, 2004). The World Health Organization Global Strategy urges countries to:

- Set national dietary and physical activity guidelines.
- Provide accurate and balanced information to consumers in order to facilitate healthy choices.
- Create health literacy and education programs.
- Set marketing and advertising restrictions, particularly protecting children.
- Mandate nutrition labeling so consumers can make healthy choices
- Regulate health claims on products.
- Change national agriculture policies to promote public health.
- Support community policies to promote physical activity through changes in the environment.
- Support school policies that promote healthy eating and physical activity.
- Consult with stakeholders, including the private sector, nongovernmental organizations, and civil society to get input on how to curtail obesity.
- Support health care providers in offering preventive services.

- Invest government budgets in surveillance, research, and evaluation.

The United Kingdom has been one of the front runners in obesity prevention efforts by adopting a multicomponent strategy to prevent obesity (Government Office for Science, 2008). They have banned marketing of foods high in fat, sugar, and salt during television programs that appeal to kids younger than 16 years. Other strategies include promoting breastfeeding, investing in making schools more healthy, increasing participation in school sports, initiating social marketing campaigns, working with the Association of Convenience Stores to promote the purchase of fruits and vegetables, investing in changes to the built environment to increase physical activity, working with employers, working with health care providers to increase access to weight management services, and creating various government departments and agencies to facilitate changes.

Many other countries and groups, such as the European Union, have developed obesity prevention strategies, with a recognition that obesity is taking a tremendous financial and human toll on our population. Hopefully, the rest of the world is watching and taking notes.

WHAT IS OBESITY COSTING US?

Obesity is tremendously costly to our society, both literally and figuratively. Financially, obese adults in the United States will incur an additional $3.47 billion in additional medical expenses annually because they were obese or overweight as children (Trasande, 2010). Although there is limited cost-effectiveness data on treating and preventing obesity (John, Wenig, & Wolfenstetter, 2010), there are some studies that have made projections about how much obesity prevention could save us. Spending $2 billion per year would be cost effective if it reduced obesity among 12-year-olds by one percentage point (Trasande, 2010). Another recent study estimated that a 1% reduction in obesity prevalence among teens in the United States would result in a decrease of $586.3 million or $73 per capita in lifetime medical costs (Wang, Denniston, Lee, Galuska, & Lowry, 2010). Imagine the kind of savings we could achieve with a more substantial reduction in prevalence!

PARTING WORDS

We did not become a country where the majority of people are overweight or obese overnight; nor did the prevalence of obesity double across the globe solely because of fast food, soda, or video games. It is the result of decades of hundreds or thousands of gradual (and sometimes sudden) changes in how our society operates that has created the current dysfunctional system that promotes unhealthy eating and inactivity. Similarly, it will take decades to restructure this system to be more conducive to health, perhaps longer, given the entrenched interests vested in maintaining the status quo. It is simply easier to put off making wide-scale changes and blame the individual, leaving it up to them to figure it out.

Reversing the obesity epidemic is at least on the global agenda. Innovative strategies are being created and tested all the time in communities, schools, workplaces, states, and countries. Maybe, by the time the sequel to this book comes out, we will have some answers to the question of "how can we effectively treat and prevent obesity?" Who knows—maybe the title of a book we write in 30 years will be, "Slaying the Dragon: How Society Conquered Obesity." It could happen. Stay tuned. In the meantime, we will leave you with some optimistic parting words from the World Health Organization (2004, p. 16):

> Changes in patterns of diet and physical activity will be gradual, and national strategies will need a clear plan for long-term and

sustained disease-prevention measures. However, changes in risk factors and in incidence of non-communicable diseases can occur quite quickly when effective interventions are made.

NOTE

[1]http://www.letsmove.gov/

REFERENCES

Anderson, J. W., Konz, E. C., Frederich, R. C., & Wood, C. L. (2001). Long-term weight-loss maintenance: A meta-analysis of US studies. *American Journal of Clinical Nutrition, 74*, 579–584.

Finucane, M. M., Stevens, G. A., Cowan, M. J., Danaei, G., Lin, J. K., Paciorek, C. J.,...Ezzati, M. (2011). National, regional, and global trends in body-mass index since 1980: Systematic analysis of health examination surveys and epidemiological studies with 960 country-years and 9.1 million participants. *Lancet, 377*, 557–567.

Government Office for Science. (2008). *Tackling obesities: Future choices, One-Year Review, October 2007–November 2008*. Retrieved February 16, 2011, from http://www.bis.gov.uk/foresight/our-work/projects/published-projects/tackling-obesities

Hodge, A. M., Dowse, G. K., & Zimmet, P. Z. (1996). Obesity in Pacific populations. *Public Health Dialog, 3*, 77–86.

International Agency for Research on Cancer. (2011). *The GloboCan Project*. Retrieved February 16, 2011, from http://globocan.iarc.fr/

International Obesity Task Force. (2011). *The global epidemic*. Retrieved February 16, 2011, from http://www.iaso.org/iotf/obesity/obesity theglobalepidemic/

John, J., Wenig, C. M., & Wolfenstetter, S. B. (2010). Recent economic findings on childhood obesity: Cost-of-illness and cost-effectiveness of interventions. *Current Opinions in Clinical Nutrition and Metabolic Care, 13*(3), 305–313.

Marks, K. (2010, December 26). Fat of the land: Nauru tops obesity league. *The Independent*. Retrieved February 16, 2011, from http://www.independent.co.uk/life-style/health-and-families/health-news/fat-of-the-land-nauru-tops-obesity-league-2169418.html

Monteiro, C. A., Conde, W. L., Lu, B., & Popkin, B. M. (2004). Obesity and inequities in health in the developing world. *International Journal of Obesity, 28*, 1181–1186.

Popkin, B. M., & Gordon-Larsen, P. (2004). The nutrition transition: Worldwide obesity dynamics and their determinants. *International Journal of Obesity, 28*, S2–S9.

Runge, C. F. (2007). Economic consequences of the obese. *Diabetes, 56*, 2668–2672.

Trasande, L. (2010). How much should we invest in preventing childhood obesity? *Health Affairs, 29*(3), 372–378.

Wang, L. Y., Denniston, M., Lee, S., Galuska, D., & Lowry, R. (2010). Long-term health and economic impact of preventing and reducing overweight and obesity in adolescence. *Journal of Adolescent Health, 46*, 467–473.

World Cancer Research Fund International. (2011). *Cancer preventability estimates for food, nutrition, body fatness, and physical activity.* Retrieved February 16, 2011, from http://www.wcrf.org/cancer_research/policy_report/preventability_estimates_food.php

World Health Organization. (2004). *Global strategy on diet, physical activity and health. WHA57.17.* Geneva, Switzerland: Author.

World Health Organization. (2011). *Obesity and overweight: Fact sheet.* Retrieved February 16, 2011, from http://www.who.int/mediacentre/factsheets/fs311/en/index.html

Index